Beyond Rice Cakes

LIST OF CONTRIBUTORS

The National Foundation for Celiac Awareness
Marla Gold
Christina Perillo
Susan Schurr
Lee Tobin
Ann Whelan

Beyond Rice Cakes

A Young Person's Guide to Cooking, Eating & Living Gluten-Free

Vanessa L. Maltin

In association with the
National Foundation for Celiac Awareness

iUniverse, Inc.
New York Lincoln Shanghai

Beyond Rice Cakes
A Young Person's Guide to Cooking, Eating & Living Gluten-Free

iUniverse books may be ordered through booksellers or by contacting:

iUniverse
2021 Pine Lake Road, Suite 100
Lincoln, NE 68512
www.iuniverse.com
1-800-Authors (1-800-288-4677)

Illustrations by Julie Hyman & Amanda Mangalavite

ISBN-13: 978-0-595-40424-7 (pbk)
ISBN-13: 978-0-595-84800-3 (ebk)
ISBN-10: 0-595-40424-3 (pbk)
ISBN-10: 0-595-84800-1 (ebk)

Printed in the United States of America

To my mom: Your love and support will forever inspire me, not only in the kitchen, but in all parts of my life. You are the most wonderful mom a girl could ever have.

To Alice Bast and Nancy Ginter at NFCA: Throughout writing this book, you've both taught me so many valuable lessons about celiac disease, but more importantly, you've taught me that keeping a positive attitude is the best way to improve my life and to make others' lives better. What you've given me is one of the greatest gifts a person could ever receive.

To the Gluten-Free Girls: You are the greatest friends a girl could ever have. I only hope that all people with celiac disease have such a wonderful support system.

Table of Contents

Foreword

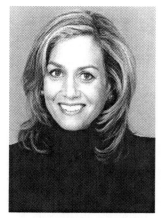

Alice Bast
Executive Director
National Foundation for Celiac Awareness

Congratulations! You are on your own! This is an exciting time in your life bringing both change and opportunity. For those of us with celiac disease, the real challenge is maintaining a gluten-free lifestyle while enjoying every moment of the life we are living.

Beyond Rice Cakes: A Young Person's Guide to Cooking, Eating & Living Gluten-Free is designed to help cross the threshold to independent living with ease, good humor and fun. We know that you will enjoy these easy-to-make recipes. Even more valuable are the tips for navigating the gluten-free waters in college, on your first job and in that new apartment after graduation.

Remember. It's all about attitude! Those diagnosed with celiac disease are so fortunate. The "cure" for our disease lies in simply eating the right foods and avoiding those that can harm us. We don't have to take pills, get shots, keep extensive records or go for treatments. Yes, we do have to read labels and ask lots of questions. But, that's it! You can even have beer and pizza that is gluten-free! With care, life can be a banquet.

The National Foundation for Celiac Awareness is dedicated to raising awareness and funds for research for celiac disease. We want to make your journey into an independent gluten-free lifestyle as easy as possible. *Beyond Rice Cakes* is a vital part of fulfilling that mission as we work to improve the quality of life of those affected by this autoimmune disease.

With best wishes for a healthy, happy and gluten-free life,

Alice

Author's Note

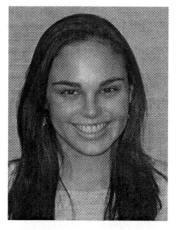

Vanessa Maltin
Diagnosed with celiac August 2004

For the first 21 years of my life I lived like any other young person. I ate pizza, sandwiches, cookies and cake and, like most other college students, welcomed my 21st birthday with a cold beer. However, unlike most of my friends who could stay out and party all night long, nearly every time I ate I got sick. We're not talking sick like I had a cold with a runny and stuffy nose. We're talking about constant diarrhea. No...let's be honest here. Explosive diarrhea that just kept flowing until there was nothing left in my stomach, but just kept coming.

Yes, I farted, much to the dismay of many of my male friends who didn't believe that girly girls actually passed gas. I had headaches all the time and what seemed like a permanent room at the George Washington University Hospital. It was a big joke among my friends about who was going to be the next one to run to the drugstore to buy me anti-diarrhea medication. I should have been the poster child for Pepto-Bismal.

For 21 years I endured constant stomachaches, migraine headaches and unexplained skin problems. I visited doctor after doctor, took several courses of steroids and experimented with every migraine medication on the market. I even showed up to my sorority formal with an IV in my arm because the doctors couldn't figure out a better way to keep me out of bed. Nothing helped.

For all of those years I was essentially poisoning myself just by eating what I thought were normal meals.

At long last I was diagnosed with celiac disease as a college student. At that moment I should have been incredibly relieved that a doctor had finally found the cause of all of my illnesses. However, my reaction was quite different. I thought that my life as I knew it had come to an end. So, I cried and complained about how I would never be able to eat like a normal person ever again.

My celiac diagnosis meant that I had to eliminate all of the delicious gluten-based products from my daily diet. There would be no more Monday night extravaganzas with my friends at the local pub for half-priced pizza and beer, and I definitely would not be ordering my favorite soy sauce-laced Chinese foods. This was a major lifestyle change for a college kid.

One of my biggest concerns was telling my friends that I could no longer eat the same foods that they could. How would I ever explain on a first date that I had to order my hamburger without the bun, not because I was trying to lose weight, but because it would make me sick? How was I going to explain that celiac isn't a horrible disease that people can catch by touching me? How would I explain that I was still normal?

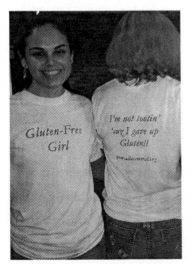

Me and my mom with our "Gluten-Free Girls" t-shirts

My mom was diagnosed with celiac disease seven years prior to me, so she knew how to manage her diet at home and I knew a little bit from watching her manage her gluten-free lifestyle. Being in college was a completely different story. I did not have a fully stocked kitchen or time between classes, working and writing for the school paper to prepare well-balanced gluten-free meals. Worst of all, none of the people around me knew what celiac disease was and I thought most people didn't want to hear about it.

Upon returning to college for my senior year, I found that the only things I could eat in my college dining hall on a regular basis were coffee, white rice and mixed nuts…meal of champions, right? Even the pre-made salads came with croutons and the fruit cups were topped with yogurt and granola. They didn't sell plain ice cream, only ice cream bars that were in some way covered with cookies, brownies or some other product containing gluten. My parents had already paid $1,000 for a meal plan that was essentially useless. I'm not going to lie…several times I cheated on my diet because it was easier than finding a gluten-free option.

At bars I constantly had to explain why I didn't want to drink beer. People would tease me, saying that I was on the "disease version of Atkins" or that I had tastes that were "too classy" to consume beer.

One night I was on a date with a seemingly great guy who nearly freaked out when I told him I couldn't eat gluten. He asked me three times if I would have a life-threatening reaction if he drank beer and ordered pasta in my presence. He thought the fumes would cause an allergic reaction. He said he didn't want to have to take me to the emergency room…classy guy right? On another date, I was asked to leave the restaurant because most of the entrees were made with gluten. That was one of the most embarrassing moments of my life.

I was depressed about my situation for about a month, but with a great deal of inspiration from my parents and the support of the National Foundation for Celiac Awareness, I decided that instead of being upset about my condition, I would be happy because for the first time in 21 years, I wasn't sick!! Imagine that. I could go an entire day without having to scramble to find a bathroom to dispense of everything I'd eaten. I could finally go to a movie without getting a headache and even better, my skin was actually clear. For the first time I was a happy and very healthy college kid.

Accepting my disease as a blessing rather than a curse was by far one of the greatest moments of my life. The realization was life altering and one I hope to share with all young people who have celiac disease.

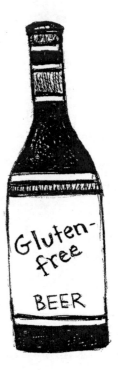

At that point I started getting excited about making gluten-free meals. I began cooking using obvious gluten-free foods and mixes that I purchased at various nutrition stores such as Whole Foods, Wegmans and the Gluten-Free Pantry. Much to my surprise, my friends seemed to love everything I made and were actually excited to learn how to cook gluten-free. Either that or they pretended to be so I would cook for them!!

As my cooking improved, my friends continued to embrace the gluten-free lifestyle and even helped me on my quest to find a bar in Washington, D.C. that served gluten-free beer and to bake my own great tasting gluten-free pizza. Beer in hand, we spent countless nights experimenting with new and fun ways to make gluten-free meals and even started calling ourselves the "Gluten-Free Girls."

After graduating from college and starting my first job, I quickly learned that living a gluten-free life in an office was no easy task. At our first company lunch, there was nothing I could eat. At my office birthday celebration I was unable to eat the delicious-looking pastries my coworkers brought because they were not gluten-free. This time I didn't get upset.

With the help of the "Gluten-Free Girls" and my mom's fantastic brownie and peanut butter cookie recipes, I quickly convinced my coworkers that gluten-free food is often as good, if not better, than traditional baked goods. Today they request my cookies and brownies for every celebration and even awarded me the "People's Choice Award" at a recent departmental bake-off. Many of those coworkers were generous enough to help with this book.

Beyond Rice Cakes: A Young Person's Guide to Cooking, Eating & Living Gluten-Free began as a binder filled with a few gluten-free recipes from my mom that sat on my kitchen countertop. With the help of my mom, my grandmother's recipe box, my closest friends and a wealth of guidance from Alice Bast and Nancy Ginter at the National Foundation for Celiac Awareness, it has turned into a priceless collection of easy-to-make recipes that any young person can master. In addition to the great-tasting recipes, the book offers young people advice from celiac disease experts and information that I wish I had known at first diagnosis: people with celiac can live healthy and happy lives.

Whether it's explaining celiac to your doctor, negotiating with your college to forgo a meal plan, talking to friends about celiac disease, dating, dining at restaurants or just learning to accept your new lifestyle, I hope that this book will let you laugh at the crazy experiences people with celiac have and realize that living a gluten-free life is not as difficult as it seems. After all, I'm not tootin' 'cuz I gave up gluten!!

Introduction

"Celiac?? Who's she? Is she contagious? Are you celiac? Is it like an STD?"

It is amazing what people who don't know about celiac will say about the disease when they encounter someone who can't eat a spinach turnover at a party. The above quote came from a seemingly nice young man I met near the mistletoe at a holiday party.

When I first heard this outrageous comment I started to laugh uncontrollably. I had no idea how anyone—especially someone at a somewhat swanky holiday party—could actually think that celiac was a sexually transmitted disease. Although the comment left me with little desire to use the mistletoe to my advantage to get a holiday kiss, I did feel the need to explain why his comment was so out of line.

Before responding to Mr. STD, I momentarily considered the deeper meaning of his comment and what it meant for my life. What if I was allergic to peanuts or was lactose intolerant? Would he have made the same comments? Probably not…because these allergies are more frequently discussed and socially accepted. Although a gluten intolerance is less talked about on a daily basis, the restrictions of celiac are in essence no different than those posed by food allergies.

There is no reason why people living with celiac disease should feel alienated, especially under the mistletoe on a happy occasion…come on, you're supposed to be kissed!! But kissing aside, it is even more important that if someone does make a stupid comment, that people with celiac are able to laugh it off and correct the misconception. As a celiac community, we must all find the motivation and courage to spread the word that not being able to eat gluten is NO BIG DEAL and will make you healthier in the long run!!

Throughout this book, I truly hope to help young people with celiac realize they can eat just as well as people who eat gluten, and empower them to show others that a gluten-free lifestyle can be easy, healthy and fun to maintain.

So, the next time someone makes a negative remark about celiac, whether it occurs at a social gathering, at work or at school, take the time to educate them and explain how great gluten-free cookies can taste…and well, if their comments don't stop, then they deserve to be left under the mistletoe with their gluten-laced spinach turnover…

Notes from the Gluten-Free Girls

Encouragement and support from my family and friends were by far the most important factors in learning to manage a gluten-free lifestyle. I was lucky that they wanted to understand my disease and help me cope with it. My best friends do not have celiac, but I quickly learned that my openness about the disease made them want to be a part of my new lifestyle. I guarantee that your friends will respond in the same way if you give them the chance.

Here are some words from my closest friends, my "Gluten-Free Girls."

Allison Goldstein

Ice cream, pizza, cookies or quiche, friendships for most college students are centered around food. At first, I thought that Vanessa not being able to eat pizza and drink beer at our weekly outings would put a damper on our social life. But over the last two years I've watched Vanessa adapt to having celiac and for the first time since I've known her, she is healthy. She has put her creativity into her cooking and together, our group of friends has adjusted to the new lifestyle and essentially become gluten-free as well…not because we feel bad, but because we like the food!!

Vanessa makes cooking fun and she works hard to keep herself healthy. She is a great example of how all people with celiac disease can live.

So, if you have celiac, take the time to do what Vanessa did with all of her friends. Talk to them about the disease. Let them know that it isn't so bad and that all it takes is a little creativity. After all, it isn't the pizza that makes you best friends…leave that responsibility up to the ice cream…or even better, make gluten-free pizza!!

Kate Ackerman

I remember going to lunch with Vanessa and some other friends after a journalism class during college. We all ordered burgers, sandwiches and pizza, but Vanessa asked for a salad without croutons. I automatically assumed she was on some sort of diet but I soon learned that she was simply trying to manage celiac disease in a life that revolved around beer and pasta.

As a person who cherishes my morning bagel, it was hard for me at first to understand and relate to Vanessa's dietary restrictions. Our friends all tried to pick restaurants where we knew she could find something to eat but we constantly found ourselves asking "does this have gluten in it?" for just about every food item.

Instead of feeling embarrassed or awkward at a party when she had to turn down a beer, Vanessa became proactive. She took the time to educate our friends about celiac and started hosting gluten-free dinner parties. With the help of her gluten-free cookies, we soon realized that living gluten-free isn't so bad and that the food actually tastes pretty good!!

Vanessa and I now live together and we rotate making dinner for each other. I look forward to her gluten-free cooking and I've become a master at finding ways to make my favorite meals into gluten-free alternatives as well. I've even learned to always read the ingredient list on packaged foods before buying them.

Our group of friends has always supported Vanessa because of her willingness to help us understand and embrace her condition. You're friends will do the same if you give them the opportunity...and if they need a little convincing, just make them chocolate fudge brownies and remind them that Tequila is naturally gluten-free!!

Expert Notes

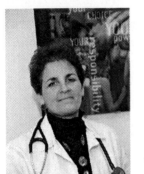

Marla Gold, M.D.
Dean, Drexel University School of Public Health

Welcome to the world of gluten-free cooking!! Using this cookbook means that you or someone you know is likely intolerant to gluten, most commonly found in wheat, barley and rye. This condition is known as celiac disease, and recent studies indicate it is quite common. Researchers estimate that 0.5 percent to 1 percent of Americans have celiac disease—up to three million people.

Celiac was once viewed by the medical community as a rare disease. Only recently did the National Institutes of Health announce that it affects millions of people. This is a serious public health issue with long-term consequences. Drexel University School of Public Health wants to raise the profile of this issue and truly stands behind National Foundation for Celiac Awareness's vital mission to improving awareness and diagnosis of celiac disease.

People with celiac disease range from babies who fail to thrive early in life due to gluten reactions that interfere with food and nutrient absorption, to teenagers and adults who have recently been diagnosed after perhaps years of gastrointestinal problems.

The disease causes chronic inflammation of the small intestine from repeated gluten consumption and can lead to poor growth and significant other problems later in life. Currently, the diagnosis is made with a blood test followed by an endoscopy, which examines and biopsies the small intestinal tissue.

Scientists are working to cure celiac disease, but until then, modifying your diet will provide the best remedy. The "treatment" for celiac disease is complete avoidance of gluten. The great news is that if you do not eat any gluten, you will feel better fast!!

In the beginning, adhering to a gluten-free diet may be challenging. You must become educated about grains, thoroughly read food labels and understand that gluten can be a hidden ingredient. Wheat comes in many forms, giving rise to over a dozen names such as kamut, spelt, bulgur and couscous—all of them forbidden.

Foods made from rye and barley are also toxic to those with celiac disease—and that includes malt which is made from barley. Hence, what begins as a directive to avoid wheat, rye and barley, can quickly grow to a long list of foods that a person with celiac cannot eat.

While the list of "no's" may be long, the list of what you can eat is much larger (and delicious) than you think!! Gluten-free food can be tasty and exciting. The safest and often tastiest way to ensure a gluten-free meal is to prepare it yourself.

Working with the National Foundation for Celiac Awareness, the "Gluten-Free Girls" have put together this incredible collection of recipes. Taking care to buy the right ingredients and learning to cook gluten-free is one of the keys to keeping healthy and avoiding problems in the future. You have the power to be gluten-free!! It may seem daunting at first, but with a little practice, you will find friends and family clamoring for your cooking!!

What is Celiac Disease??

Celiac disease is an inherited autoimmune disease that damages the small intestines, interferes with absorption of food and then triggers other seemingly unrelated health conditions. Celiac affects about one in every 133 Americans, most of whom are misdiagnosed because their symptoms mirror other conditions such as Irritable Bowel Syndrome, anemia, psychological stress and diarrhea. If left untreated, celiac can lead to infertility, osteoporosis, lymphoma, depression and neurological disorders. It is more common than Alzheimer's, Type 1 diabetes and multiple sclerosis.

Facts about celiac:

- 2.96 million Americans across all races, ages and genders suffer from celiac.
- 97% of celiacs are undiagnosed or misdiagnosed.
- 9 years is the average time a person waits to be correctly diagnosed with celiac.
- 17% of celiac patients have an immediate family member who also suffers from celiac.
- There are currently NO pharmaceutical cures for celiac, underscoring the need for further research in the field.
- A 100% gluten-free diet is the only existing treatment for celiac today.
- 500,000 new celiac diagnoses are expected to occur in the next five years.
- $5,000 to $12,000 is the average cost of misdiagnosis per person/per year of celiac, not including lost work time.

How to recognize if you have celiac disease??

Common Symptoms

- Chronic diarrhea
- Constipation
- Gas
- Recurring abdominal bloating
- Weight loss/weight gain
- Fatigue
- Bone or joint pain
- Osteoporosis, osteopenia
- Muscle cramps
- Pale sores inside mouth
- Skin irritation
- Foul-smelling or fatty stool
- Tingling numbness in legs
- Tooth discoloration or loss of enamel

What to do if you think you have celiac disease...

1. Schedule an appointment with your physician for a blood test called the Celiac Panel. This test includes the following analysis: anti-endomysial antibody (IgA EMA) and anti-gliadin antibody (IgA & IgG), and tissue transglutaminase (tTG IgA).

2. If the blood test results are positive or your physician suspects you have celiac disease, you should schedule an appointment with a gastroenterologist to undergo an endoscopy and a small intestine tissue biopsy that will show damaged villi in the small intestine—the "Gold Standard" for diagnosing celiac disease.

How Do I Treat Celiac Disease??

To date, the only treatment for celiac disease is to follow a STRICT gluten-free diet for life. This means avoiding all foods that contain gluten (wheat, barley and rye). Eliminating gluten will allow the damaged small intestines to heal and reduce the risk of developing celiac-related conditions.

Tips for managing a gluten-free lifestyle:

1. Maintain a life-long gluten-free diet
2. Educate family, friends and community about celiac
3. Identify and treat personal nutritional deficiencies
4. Join a celiac support group
5. Follow up with a physician regularly for life
6. Consult with a skilled dietician

What NOT to eat:

- Wheat (in all forms including Kamut, spelt, semolina, farina, einkorn, bulgar, couscous and triticale)
- Rye
- Barley (in all forms including malt, malt syrup, malt extract and malt flavorings)

Hidden sources of gluten in common products:

Prescription medications

Lip gloss, Chapstick, lipstick

Malt or malt flavoring

Dairy substitutes

Licorice

Soy sauce

Salad dressing, soups, gravies

Seasonings

Dextrin

Malted beverages

Vitamins

Playdough

**See definitions for details

What Can I Eat??

Safe Starches:

Amaranth
Modified tapioca starch
Buckwheat
Corn
Rice and wild rice
Potato and tubers
Quinoa
Tapioca
Teff
Arrowroot
Sorghum
Montina
Millet
Ragi
Chickpea
Lentil
Soy

Definitions

Provided by *Gluten-Free Living,* a full-color magazine that for 10 years has published well-researched articles and lifestyle materials to improve the lives of those who follow a gluten-free diet.

Amaranth
A healthy gluten-free plant similar to grains.

Buckwheat
Despite the name, buckwheat is a fruit so it's gluten-free. It is no more likely to be contaminated than any grain, but it is sometimes mixed with wheat flour, so you can't automatically assume all buckwheat products are gluten-free. Always read the label. Buckwheat is nutritious and adds variety to the gluten-free diet.

Caramel color
According to the Food and Drug Administration Code of Federal Regulations (CFR), caramel color can be made from barley malt. But US companies use corn because it makes a better product.

Citric Acid
This ingredient is gluten-free.

Dextrin
According to the FDA Code of Federal Regulations (CFR), dextrin can be made from corn, potato, arrowroot, rice, tapioca or wheat. Major dextrin-producing companies in the US say they use corn. However, imported dextrin could be made from wheat.

Flavors

Flavors are tricky. It is often difficult to find out what is in a flavoring. But according to the Flavor Extract Manufacturers Association, gluten-containing grains are rarely used in flavoring except in meat products and products that contain meat.

Hydrolyzed vegetable protein or Hydrolyzed Plant Protein?

These ingredients should not be confusing. Ten years ago the FDA said food processors had to identify the vegetable or plant by name. So, food labels might list "hydrolyzed wheat protein" (unsafe) or "hydrolyzed soy protein" (safe), for example.

Malt

Although there is a slight chance that "malt" is made from corn, it is almost always derived from barley so it contains gluten. Malt extract, malt syrup and malt flour are made from barley. So is malt vinegar and it is not distilled, so it could contain gluten.

Maltodextrin

When labeled as "maltodextrin" in the US, this ingredient must be made from corn, potato or rice but not wheat. Confusion comes from the name. Malt is usually made from barley and dextrin can be made from wheat. But maltodextrin is gluten-free. Recently there has been some evidence that wheat might be used to produce maltodextrin. If it is, the label will specifically say "wheat maltodextrin" or "maltodextrin (wheat)."

Mono and diglycerides

Mono and diglycerides are fats and therefore gluten-free. But there has been concern that a gluten-containing carrier might be used to make them perform as the food processor wants. Research indicates that this rarely happens and when it does, the carrier should be declared.

Oats

When wheat was identified as a cause of celiac disease, rye, barley and oats were also included on the list of toxic grains. But in recent years, several well respected research studies strongly suggest that oats do not belong on the list. However, growing conditions and the appearance of the grain make it very likely that oats are easily contaminated with wheat. Therefore US celiac experts have not yet approved oats for the gluten-free diet.

Oat gum

Oat gum is rarely used as an ingredient. But when it is, it should be gluten-free. Gluten is a protein and oat gum is made from the carbohydrate portion of oats. Moreover, researchers now say oats are gluten-free.

Quinoa

An ancient grain-like plant from South America that is gluten-free. It is no more likely to be contaminated with gluten than any other gluten-free plant. Quinoa is nutritious and adds variety to the gluten-free diet.

Soy Sauce

Some (but not all) contain wheat. Read the label.

Spelt

Spelt is a form of wheat. In the past, some spelt producers have labeled their product as "gluten-free," which is incorrect. Although those who are *allergic* to wheat may be able to tolerate spelt, it is still a form of wheat and therefore not gluten-free.

Spices and Seasonings

Pure spices are gluten-free. Bottled spices often contain something to keep the spice free flowing. Usually it's silicon dioxide, which is gluten-free. If a spice container does not have a list of ingredients on the label, the only thing it contains is the spice indicated.

Seasonings have not been defined by the FDA and therefore could contain anything. Sometimes the contents of a seasoning are included on the label in parenthesis.

Starch

On a *food* label, starch always indicates cornstarch. That's the only certainty. Although usually made from corn, modified food starch can be made from wheat. In *pharmaceuticals*, both starch and modified food starch can be made from wheat.

Vanilla

Vanilla and vanilla extract are gluten-free.

Vinegar

Distilled vinegar is gluten-free and has always been gluten-free. There is no evidence that suggests vinegar might be dangerous for those who follow the gluten-free diet. The only vinegar to avoid is malt vinegar, which is not distilled.

Wheat Starch

Wheat starch is wheat with the gluten washed out. A special grade of wheat starch is permitted on the gluten-free diet in some European countries, but it is not permitted here in the US. That's because the washing process is rarely complete and wheat starch usually contains residual gluten.

Yeast

All brand-name packaged yeasts sold in the US are gluten-free. Autolyzed yeast in a food product is generally considered gluten-free. Brewers yeast, when it's a by-product of beer, is not considered gluten-free. Brewers yeast nutritional supplements, however, can be made from either brewer's yeast or sugar. If made from sugar, they are gluten-free.

Gluten-Free Cooking Substitutes:

Brown Rice Flour

Corn Flour

Cornstarch

Guar Gum

Modified Tapioca Starch

Potato Flour

Potato Starch Flour

Soy Flour

Sweet Rice Flour

Tapioca Flour

White Rice Flour

Xanthan Gum

Gluten-Free Measurement Conversions

For each cup of wheat flour substitute:

1 cup cornmeal

1 cup corn flour

3/4 cup rice flour

1 1/4 cups soy flour

1 cup modified tapioca starch

2/3 cup potato starch

1/2 cup soy flour + 1/2 cup corn starch

1/2 cup soy flour + 1/2 cup potato flour

1/2 cup rice flour + 1/2 cup soy flour

Where Do I Find Gluten-Free Food??

Dining Out:

We all have horror stories…one of mine occurred while I was trying to order a gluten-free meal at a Malaysian restaurant in Washington, D.C. I was on a majorly hot date and the guy had been telling me about this new restaurant for days. The date seemed to be going great until I tried to order dinner. I asked our waiter if the chicken in the dish I was ordering was breaded with flour. He responded by asking me if I was allergic to gluten.

At first I was a little bit excited that he knew about the gluten intolerance. However, my excitement quickly disappeared when he asked us to leave the restaurant because I was a "liability." That night I cried, complained to my family and friends, and considered never dining out again.

Although this experience was horrible, it was isolated; to date I've had almost entirely positive experiences eating at restaurants. I've even found restaurants that have entire gluten-free menus or that will convert any item on the menu to a gluten-free alternative, such as Shanghai Garden in Washington, D.C. and Risotteria in New York City. I just have to remember that it is my job to explain my condition and help the waiters, waitresses and cooks understand how to prepare my meal with gluten-free ingredients.

My one embarrassing night out was significant because it helped me realize how little the public knows about celiac disease.

Here are a few tips for raising awareness and having a great night out:

• Call the restaurant ahead of time (preferably not during peak hours) and ask if they have gluten-free options on their menu or if they are able to adapt their offerings to be gluten-free.

• Bring your own gluten-free soy sauce and salad dressings

• Order your salad without croutons

• Order a plain piece of meat or fish

• Ask to substitute gluten-based side dishes with steamed vegetables, rice or potatoes

National Restaurant Chains with Gluten-Free Options:

Bone Fish Grill
www.bonefishgrill.com
866-880-2226

Boston Market
www.bostonmarket.com
800-365-7000

Chick-Fil-A
www.chick-fil-a.com
866-CFA-2040

Carrabba's Italian Grill
www.carrabbas.com

Dairy Queen
www.dairyqueen.com
952-830-0200

Don Pablo's
www.donpablos.com
800-372-2567

Legal Sea Foods
www.legalseafoods.com

McDonald's
www.mcdonalds.com
800-244-6227

Mitchell's Fish Market
www.cameronmitchell.com
614-621-3663

Outback Steakhouse
www.outback.com

P.F. Changs
www.pfchangs.com
866-PFCHANG

Red Lobster
www.redlobster.com
800-562-7837

Texas Roadhouse
www.texasroadhouse.com
800-TEX-ROAD

Wendy's
www.wendys.com
614-764-3100

Where to buy gluten-free food:

Andronico's Market
www.andronicos.com

Hannaford Supermarkets
www.hannaford.com

Mollie Stones
www.molliestones.com

Trader Joes
www.traderjoes.com

Wegmans
www.wegmans.com

Whole Foods
www.wholefoods.com

Gluten-free specialty stores:

Aunt Candice
www.auntcandicefoods.com

The Gluten-Free Cookie Jar
www.glutenfreecookiejar.com

Gluten-Free Mall
www.glutenfreemall.com

The Gluten-free Market
www.glutenfreemarket.com

Gluten-Free Pantry
www.glutenfree.com

Gluten Smart
www.store.glutensmart.com

Gluten Solutions
www.glutensolutions.com

Glutino
www.glutino.com

My Gluten-free Store
www.myglutenfreestore.com

Gluten-free wedding cakes:

So…you don't want a rice cake wedding cake?? Although rice cakes are the staple of most celiac's diets, there are few young people who would actually want their wedding cake made out of the crunchy, flaky cakes. Don't worry, many bakeries across the country actually offer gluten-free varieties…

Below is a list of several bakeries in big cities, small cities, and even in the middle-of-no-where that offer gluten-free wedding cake selections.

CALIFORNIA
Crave Bakery
San Francisco, CA
415-826-7187
Web Site: www.cravebakery.org
Email: info@cravebakery.org

Dessert by Design
San Diego, CA 92159
619-374-2101

Maggie's Bakery
6530 Lankershim Boulelvard #L
North Hollywood, CA 91606
818-506-6265

ILLINOIS
Crème de la Crème Wedding Cakes
1507 East 53rd Street., #206
Chicago, IL
773-363-1650

IOWA
Specialty Cakes & More
712 North 4th Street
Grimes, IA 50111
515-986-4630
Web Site: www.specialtycakes.net/glutenfree.htm

HAWAII
Sweet Marie's
PO Box 98
Kapaa, HI 96746
808-823-8446
Email: sweetmaries@hawaiian.net
Web Site: www.sweetmarieskauai.com

MASSACHUSETTS
Hippie Chick Bakery
11 Elm Street
Amesbury, MA 01913
978-388-6644
Web Site: www.hippiechickbakery.com

The Organic Gourmet
58 Schoolhouse Road
Amherst, MA 01002
413-259-1695
Email: lescerier@aol.com
Web Site: www.members.aol.com/lescerier

MICHIGAN
Carlson Catering Company
Belleville, MI
734-699-8100
Email: food@carlsoncatering.com
Web Site: www.carlsoncatering.com

Celiac Specialties
48411 Jefferson
Chesterfield Twp, MI 48047
586-598-8180
Email: Contact-Us@CeliacSpecialties.com
Web Site: www.celiacspecialties.com

NEW YORK
TriBakery-Manhattan
186 Franklin Street
Manhattan, NY 10013
212-431-1114

Magnolia Bakery
401 Bleecker Street
New York, NY 10014-2452
212-462-2572

Happy Happy Happy
157 Allen Street
New York, NY 10002
212-254-4088

The Alternative Baker
35 Broadway
Kingston, NY 12401
845-331-5517
Email: NYBaker@aol.com
Web Site: www.lemoncakes.com

NEW JERSEY
Wildflowers
Bridgeton, New Jersey
(856) 459-3515
Email: lori@wildflowersbylori.com
Web Site: www.wildflowersbylori.com

NORTH CAROLINA
Good Taste Cake Designs, LLC.
Durham, NC
919-489-5778
Email: gtcd@aol.com
Web Site: www.goodtastecakedesigns.com

West End Bakery and Café
757 Haywood Road
West Asheville, NC
828-252-WEST
Web Site: www.onhaywood.com/westend-bakery/

OHIO
Chocolate Emporium
14486 Cedar Road
Cleveland, Ohio 44121
(216) 382-0140
1-888-CHOCLAT

OREGON
Piece of Cake Bakery
8306 Southeast 17th Street
Portland, OR 97202-7307
(503) 234-9445
Email: sales@pieceofcakebakery.net
Web Site: www.pieceofcakebakery.net

VIRGINIA
Hungarian Bakery
1230 Templeton Circle
Earlysville, VA 22936
434-973-8863
Email: hunbakery@adelphia.net
Web Site: www.hungarianbakery.com

WASHINGTON
Kaili's Kitchen
In Firdale Village
9711 Firdale Avenue
Edmonds, WA 98020
206-542-1462 or
877-664-5883

Covering increased cost of food:

Yes…gluten-free food is more expensive, but buying gluten-free varieties does not have to break the bank. Here are a few ideas for keeping your costs down:

• Shop around. Visit a variety of stores in your area to compare prices. You may find that some stores sell gluten-free products for significantly lower prices. Smaller, non-chain stores tend to have lower prices and will often order specialty foods for you.

• Buy in bulk and store. This saves on traveling expenses, and sometimes shipping expenses if flat fees are charged. A separate freezer may also help if you have the space.

• A local support group may purchase a case of food and divide the contents between its members. This gives you the chance to experiment with new foods without bearing the full cost of shipping or purchasing a large quantity of items that you may end up not liking.

Gluten-free beer:

Giving up beer can be incredibly difficult for young people, especially those who frequently visit bars. Although most bars do not keep gluten-free varieties on tap, there are many distributors nationwide where you can order your own supply. Also check with your local liquor store because they may be able to negotiate a lower price.

Ramapo Valley Brewery
www.ramapovalleybrewery.com

Bard's Tale Beer
www.bardsbeer.com

New Grist
www.newgrist.com

Green's Discovery
www.glutenfreebeers.co.uk

Nick Stafford's Hambleton Ales
www.hambletonales.co.uk

Fine Ale Club
www.ale4home.co.uk/fine_ale_club.htm

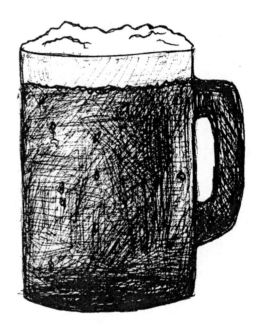

How Do I Manage My Gluten-Free Diet??

Keeping a positive attitude:

Keeping a smile on your face is often hard to do when you are constantly worrying about keeping gluten out of your diet. At times it seems like everything is on the do-not-eat list. However, getting depressed about celiac disease makes coping with the condition even more difficult. So…instead of crying, try smiling and channeling your energy toward figuring out a routine that works for you.

The first step is to remember that celiac disease is NOT THE END OF THE WORLD!! It is just as if you had any other food allergy, like millions of people worldwide. Our "allergy" isn't as well known…so start talking about it. Tell everyone you know about the condition, because they, too, might have it and not yet know. Plus, the more you talk about the disease the more people will accept it as a common digestive disorder that is NO BIG DEAL!!

Create a daily plan for managing your diet. Eat breakfast at home so you can personally ensure your meal has no gluten. Taking a homemade lunch to work or school is generally the best method for eliminating gluten. If you do plan to dine out during the day, try to buy food from places you're familiar with to limit gluten exposure. Cook dinner at home, or if you go out, call ahead to make sure the menu includes gluten-free options.

Always carry a gluten-free snack with you when you leave home. Try purchasing gluten-free snack bars from any one of the gluten-free vendors listed throughout this book. This way you will never be without something safe to eat.

Having even the simplest plan in place will help you prevent being without something to eat. You will always feel secure going out because you will be prepared and healthy. You are the only one who can make having celiac a positive experience. Get out there and be active!!

Talking to your physician:

Although celiac disease is VERY common, many physicians still consider the disease a "rare childhood condition." This is a very common misconception that must be corrected.

One way to inform your doctor is to bring him or her published information on celiac disease. If you see an article about celiac in the newspaper, cut it out and send it to your doctor. Showing him or her published documents will reinforce the fact that celiac is a real disease that affects millions of people around the world.

Another option is contacting your local celiac support group and asking for recommendations for doctors who specialize in gastrointestinal issues. They can point you to physicians who understand the disease and can help you manage your daily life.

Once again, here are the appropriate tests for accurately diagnosing celiac disease. Make sure your physician prescribes the correct test, because there is often confusion:

1. Schedule an appointment with your primary care physician for a blood test called: The Celiac Panel, which includes the anti-endomysial antibody (IgA EMA) and anti-gliadin antibody (IgA & IgG), and tissue transglutaminase (tTG IgA).

2. If the blood test results are positive or your physician suspects you have celiac disease, you should schedule an appointment with a gastroenterologist to undergo an endoscopy and a small intestine tissue biopsy that will show damaged villi in the small intestine—the "Gold Standard" for diagnosing celiac disease.

In the workplace:

The best way to get your coworkers to understand a gluten-free lifestyle is to cook for them. Many gluten-free foods taste astronomically better than their non-gluten-free counterparts. For example, many of the dessert recipes produce sinfully delicious treats and most of the meals, salads and snacks taste EXACTLY the same.

A little side story...

My first job after college was as a health care reporter for a daily publication. One would think that people working at a health care organization would have at least heard of celiac disease. This was not the case.

On my first day of work the career management department planned a welcome lunch where they served sandwiches, pasta salad and cookies for dessert…there was not one thing I could eat unless I picked the meat, cheese and vegetables out of the sandwiches and risked contamination. I was very hungry that day. Sadly, I did not say anything to the people who put on the lunch about the selection of food.

Two weeks later my department held a birthday celebration for me and again I was unable to eat any of the tasty treats they brought in. Because I was the birthday girl, people were very curious as to why I was not eating any of the food. This time I explained to them that I had celiac disease and what it entailed.

After bringing numerous types of brownies, cookies and other gluten-free goodies to various department events, they have in a way become a novelty. My coworkers always insist that I make my "famous peanut butter cookies" and brownies.

One of the most amazing experiences I've had since being diagnosed with celiac disease has been watching my coworkers learn about celiac and eventually come to embrace it. Any time there is an article in the paper about celiac, by 9 a.m. I have several copies waiting in my e-mail inbox.

My coworkers are so wonderful that many of them took the time to convert their favorite recipes into gluten-free alternatives and submit them for this cookbook.

We're all busy people and while all offices may not take to grasping a gluten-free way of life like mine did, it is up to you to take the first steps. If you know there is an upcoming office function, take the time to speak with the person planning it to make sure there are gluten-free varieties of food.

Most importantly, though, explain celiac disease to your coworkers and cook for them!! They will get hooked!!

Tips for going to parties:

•If you know the host/hostess…call ahead and ask what they are serving. Make sure they know you cannot eat gluten.
•Offer to bring a gluten-free dish. Your friends will try the food you bring and most likely will have no idea it is even gluten-free.
•Eat a snack before you go

•Pick and choose lighter fare while socializing such as fresh fruit or vegetables

•ENJOY!!

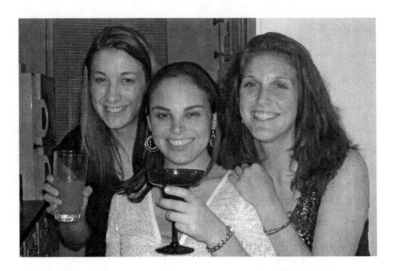

Gluten-Free Girls drinking tequila! Remember,
tequila is naturally gluten-free!

Foods to eat on the run:

Always keep energy bars, trail mix, nuts, and/or gluten-free crackers in your car, gym bag, desk, briefcase, pocketbook…just in case. Most markets listed throughout the book sell gluten-free snacks that stay fresh for long periods of time and are safe to keep with you at all times.

Traveling tips:

ALWAYS plan ahead!! Call the facility where you are staying at and explain your dietary requirements so that they have time to prepare for your arrival. Airlines are generally very helpful with arranging gluten-free meals. However, just in case, always carry trail mix, crackers, nuts, fruit or energy bars with you.

Before you leave, it's also a good idea to search the Internet for local celiac support groups, which may have lists of restaurants and food stores that accommodate gluten-free patrons.

Petitioning to forgo a college meal plan:

Moving away from home? Making new friends? Wondering how you're ever going to pay back all of those student loans? Going away to college can be difficult enough on its own, but without the comfort of private kitchens and home-cooked food, college students with celiac are often found wandering around student unions looking for something they can eat besides prepackaged garden salads that may or may not have been made with croutons. With the help of the recipes in this book and a community kitchen, if you are a student with celiac disease, you will not have to starve until Thanksgiving break.

At many universities, students living in campus residence halls are required to purchase expensive meal plans when they sign their housing contracts; often times students are unaware that these contracts are intertwined. Though they serve the practical purpose of ensuring that students living in dorms that do not have private kitchens eat, they may be restrictive for gluten-intolerant coeds. Furthermore, most universities do not easily waive the meal plan requirement.

At some privately funded universities, students are required to partake in meal plans. Students attending these schools should consult their billing services departments to petition for necessary adjustments.

Public universities may offer slightly more flexibility. One public university asks students with special diets not to live in campus housing. If a student at this school develops a disease such as celiac while living in campus housing, he or she may have to submit to additional medical testing by the university to verify the disease and eventually waive the meal plan requirement. Another publicly funded school appoints dieticians for students with special dietary needs to find ways to make the meal plan work for them.

Since meal plans and requirement policies vary from school to school, here are some handy tips for navigating your university:

• **Do your homework.** Research the university that you plan to attend. Often, their websites are great places to start. Find out what the required meal plans are, and what they offer that can be included in a gluten-free diet. If you still have questions about meal plans, call your school's department of dining services, or equivalent department. Do not to sign any housing contracts until you know the policies, as these contracts may be combined with meal plans.

• **Find out who is in charge.** Cutting through a university's red tape can be made easier if you get to know administrators. By calling your school's billing center and explaining celiac disease, they may be able to release you from your meal plan obligation, or work with you to create an altered meal plan more suitable to your needs.

• **Take good notes.** Depending on your university's administrative structure, you may get referred to a few different departments. Make sure to document every conversation you have, including who you spoke with, the date of the conversation, and what he or she told you. By keeping good records, your university administrators will see that you mean business.

• **Be firm.** Remember that you are a customer at your university, so it is the administrator's job to cater to your needs. Be unyielding in your refusal to pay a significant amount of money for gluten-laced food. Although university officials may at first try to persuade you that it is not possible to get out of a meal plan, with patience and conviction, you will find that where there is a will, there is a gluten-free way!!

Chef's Notes

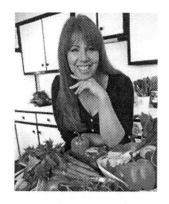

Christina Pirello

Emmy Award winning *TV personality and best-selling author, "Cooking the Whole Foods Way"*

My mom was one of the finest cooks I have ever met, and I was always hanging out with her in the kitchen. I couldn't reach the counter, so for my fourth birthday my dad made a stool, and my mom gave me this little tiny paring knife, and I got started. My mom was always so happy in the kitchen. It was the place where the whole family gathered, and it was a place I knew great joy came from. My mother baked every day. I grew up in a house where cooking wasn't a chore that you had to get through. It was just part of the daily routine.

Filled with inspiration from my mom, I began my cooking show, *Christina Cooks*. With over 140 episodes under my belt, the show delivers the information that Americans want and need to hear about maintaining a healthy daily diet. In light of the health crises we face as a nation, I take the viewer by the hand and make healthy eating fun, delicious and easy to accomplish.

As an off-shoot of my cooking show, my husband and I own a travel business. We organize holidays for people who want to continue their commitment to health even while on vacation. We organize tours of Europe, scuba trips to the Caribbean and retreats in the United States. My staff and I prepare meals to keep our guests sated and healthy. The challenges of cooking in varying locales can be exciting and daunting.

Several years ago, we received a call from a potential guest who had concerns about the food he needed for his health condition, celiac disease, and had very specific needs in order to maintain his health. I confess to having the same reactions as many chefs would, even in my line of work of healthy cooking. At first, I felt so sorry for him; no gluten seemed like an awful fate to me. And then I thought about the challenges I would face while trying to prepare special meals within the context of serving the needs of 28 other guests for three daily meals during a 10-day vacation. I admit to feeling a bit vexed over the whole thing.

I did some research to see what our guest would need to maintain his gluten-free diet and discovered that I faced the most wonderful challenge; there was so much creativity to be considered when cooking without wheat, barley and rye. I developed recipes that could work for the entire group and with the exception of a few desserts and pasta dishes, was able to feed the entire party in the same delicious manner as my special guest. There was no extra work and everyone loved the gourmet foods we were able to prepare. No one could even tell that one guest's food was gluten-free.

While celiac disease is not without its challenges, I am here to tell you that cooking gluten-free meals need not mean a diet that is dull and grim, but can be decadent, enlivening, creative and most of all, delicious!! So, head to the kitchen and fix yourself a gluten-free feast!!

Gluten-Free Girls Recipe Contest

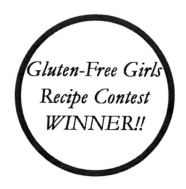

*Gluten-Free Girls
Recipe Contest
WINNER!!*

To compile the most delicious collection of gluten-free recipes, people with celiac disease and their supporters submitted recipes they thought were the tastiest and easiest to make. People from every corner of the United States submitted recipes and, while it would be fitting to recognize all of them as winners, after several rounds of taste testing there were four recipes that were the very best.

The winning recipes are featured at the beginning of their respective sections and labeled as a "Gluten-Free Recipe Contest Winner." Other recipes that were submitted are designated with the cook's name. The contest participants graciously granted permission to reprint their recipes in *Beyond Rice Cakes*.

Abby Gooding	Amanda Klein*	Brandi Hight
Brenda Ferrer	Danene Gooding	Danny Tobias

Diana Hocker   Elaine R. Grabar   Erin Smith*
Jocelyn Robbins   Karina Allrich   Laura Moore
Lianne Woolley*   Marty Bryant   Maureen Stanley*
Mike McHenry   Miriam Berg   Sophie Silver
Sylvia Chernow   Thelma Rodin   Stephanie Comeau

* denotes recipe contest winner

Getting Started

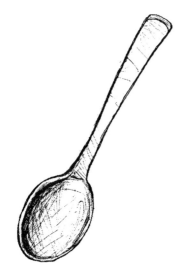

Important things to remember before cooking...

ALWAYS wash your hands.

ALWAYS cook on a clean surface. After cutting meat or poultry, wipe your work surface clean with hot soapy water.

ALWAYS double-check labels to ensure food items are gluten-free.

ALWAYS remember to set kitchen timer when putting food in the oven.

NEVER put used utensils, or anything with other food on it into a jar of condiments. Take out amount needed and put it in a separate dish or measuring cup. An easy way to prevent contamination is to purchase products that come in squeeze bottles.

NEVER leave the stove unattended.

NEVER leave dishrag or plastic bag near oven or stove.

NEVER put foil or other metal in the microwave.

Measurement Conversions

1 Tablespoon (Tblsp) = 3 Teaspoons (Tsp)

1/4 cup = 4 Tblsp

2 Tblsp = 1/2 Ounce

1 cup = 1/2 Pint

4 cups = 1 Quart

4 Quarts = 16 Ounces

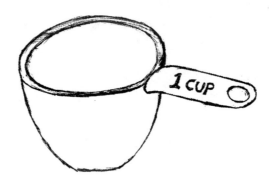

Measurement Abbreviations

Tablespoon = Tblsp

Teaspoon = Tsp

Package = pkg

Ounce = oz

Pound = lb

CAUTION

Remember to always check labels to ensure products are GLUTEN-FREE

Snacks & Finger Foods

Seven Layer Dip*
Crispy Taco Dip
Spinach Artichoke Dip
Nachos*
Sour Cream Ranch Dip
Black Bean Dip
Fruit Dip Sensation*
Peanut Butter Pumpkin Spread
Veggie Platter*
Homemade Hummus
Hummus Plate
Mini Mozzarella Skewers
Marinated Mushrooms
Raw Mushroom Surprise
Stuffed Mushrooms

Cheesy Garlic Wedges
Baked Brie & Jelly
Mango Salsa
Avocado & Corn Salsa*
Guacamole*
Ants on a Log*
Celery & Cream Cheese*
Easy Quesadillas*
Chewy Granola Bars
Cheese Plate*
Golden Potatoes
Popcorn Balls
Cornbread
Banana Roll-Up
White Bean Dip

*denotes easy to make

Maureen's Seven-Layer Dip
* Submitted by Maureen Stanley

2 pints sour cream
1/2 head shredded lettuce
2 bags shredded cheese
1 jar salsa
1 can sliced black olives
1 can sliced green olives
3 large tomatoes diced
1 bag corn tortilla chips

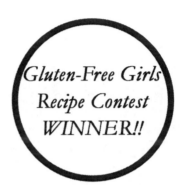

Gluten-Free Girls Recipe Contest WINNER!!

1) Spread the sour cream in the bottom of a 9 x 13-inch dish.

2) Layer the shredded cheese to completely cover sour cream.

3) Continue adding a layer of shredded lettuce, salsa, black olives, green olives and tomatoes. The final layer will be the remaining bag of shredded cheese.

4) Serve with tortilla chips.

**OPTIONAL: For more variety, consider adding a layer of taco meat, shredded chicken, beans or jalapeño peppers.

Snacks & Finger Foods

Beyond Rice Cakes

Crispy Taco Dip

8 oz cream cheese
8 oz sour cream
1 pkg taco seasoning mix
Shredded lettuce
Diced tomatoes
Diced green onions
Shredded cheddar cheese

1) Mix cream cheese, sour cream and taco seasoning mix together in small bowl.

2) Spoon into serving bowl.

3) Top with shredded lettuce, diced tomatoes, diced green onions and shredded cheddar cheese.

4) Serve with tortilla chips.

Snacks & Finger Foods

Brandi's Spinach Artichoke Dip
Submitted by Brandi Hight

1 (10 oz) package frozen chopped spinach
2 (13 3/4 oz) cans artichoke hearts
1/2 cup mayonnaise
1/2 cup sour cream
1 cup freshly grated parmesan cheese
1 cup grated Pepper Jack cheese
Dash of hot sauce to taste
Salsa or pico de gallo for garnish

1) Preheat the oven to 350 degrees.
2) Grease a casserole dish with nonstick spray.
3) Heat the spinach in a microwave oven on high for 5 minutes and squeeze dry.
4) Drain the artichoke hearts and coarsely chop in a food processor. If you do not have access to a food processor, chop artichoke hearts into small 1/2-inch pieces.
5) Combine all of the ingredients (including hot sauce) except the Jack cheese in a large bowl. Stir well.
6) Scrape into the prepared casserole dish and sprinkle the Jack cheese on top.
7) Bake for 30 minutes. Serve immediately with tortilla chips, carrots or celery.
8) Garnish with salsa or pico de gallo.

Honorable mention for Diana Hocker's Spinach Artichoke Dip

Snacks & Finger Foods

Beyond Rice Cakes

Nachos

Corn chips (enough to accommodate everyone eating)
1 cup grated cheese
1/2 cup salsa

*Optional: refried or black beans, taco meat, sour cream, guacamole

1) Preheat oven to BROIL setting.

2) Spread chips on piece of foil.

3) Cover with grated cheese.

4) Broil until cheese is melted.

5) Serve with salsa.

OPTIONAL: add favorite beans or taco meat to chips before broiling. Garnish with salsa, sour cream and guacamole.

Snacks & Finger Foods

Sour Cream Ranch Dip

1/2 cup gluten-free ranch salad dressing
1/2 cup sour cream
1 teaspoon Italian seasoning
2 teaspoon garlic powder

1)   Mix all ingredients together in small mixing bowl.

2)   Chill for about an hour before serving.

3)   Serve with raw vegetables or gluten-free crackers.

Beyond Rice Cakes

Black Bean Dip

1 (8 oz) can of black beans
1 cup shredded mozzarella, Monterey Jack or cheddar cheese
1 avocado
1 tomato
1/2 cup sour cream

1) Pour black beans into microwave-safe dish.

2) Heat for about 1 minute. Stir.

3) Chop tomato into small pieces.

4) Stir tomatoes and sour cream into black beans.

5) Sprinkle cheese on top.

6) Slice avocado and use to garnish serving dish.

7) Serve with corn chips.

Snacks & Finger Foods

Fruit Dip Sensation

1 (8 oz.) pkg soft cream cheese
2 Tablespoons orange juice
1 jar marshmallow fluff

1) Stir all ingredients together.

2) Refrigerate until ready to serve.

3) Serve with fresh fruit.

Snacks & Finger Foods

Beyond Rice Cakes

Peanut Butter Pumpkin Spread

3/4 cup peanut butter
3/4 cup canned pumpkin
3/4 cup brown sugar
1/2 teaspoon vanilla

1) Combine all of the ingredients.

2) Serve with bite-sized sliced apples, bananas and other fruit.

Snacks & Finger Foods

Veggie Platter

4 carrots
1 green pepper
1 red pepper
1 yellow pepper
1 orange pepper
1 head of broccoli
1 bunch of celery

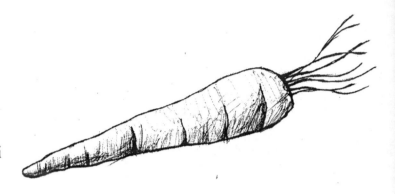

1) Slice all vegetables into bite-sized pieces and arrange on a plate.

2) Serve with favorite dip or spread.

Snacks & Finger Foods

Beyond Rice Cakes

Homemade Hummus

1(8 oz) can chickpeas
2 Tablespoon olive oil
2 teaspoon minced garlic
Dash lemon juice

1) In mixing bowl mash together chickpeas, olive oil, garlic and lemon juice until mixture is smooth.

2) Serve chilled with gluten-free crackers or vegetables.

Hummus Platter

1 container of hummus or make your own
1 package gluten-free crackers
Assortment of vegetables (Veggie Platter)

1) Arrange all ingredients nicely on a platter.

Snacks & Finger Foods

Mini Mozzarella Skewers
* Submitted by Amanda Klein

1-2 cartons cherry/grape tomatoes
1 1/2 cups fresh basil
1-2 pkg of fresh mozzarella balls
2-3 Tablespoon balsamic vinegar
1-2 cloves of chopped garlic
1 pkg of toothpicks

1) Wash tomatoes and basil and pat dry.

2) Break basil leaves off stems and set aside.

3) Take toothpicks and begin layering mozzarella, basil and tomato on each toothpick.

4) Repeat layering until you have filled appetizer tray and or have a suitable amount for your group.

5) Lastly, drizzle balsamic mixture over the mini skewers and serve.

Beyond Rice Cakes

Marinated Mushrooms

2 lbs fresh mushrooms, washed and sliced
2 cups olive oil
2 cups vinegar
1 cup water
6 cloves garlic
1/2 teaspoon oregano
1/4 teaspoon salt
1/4 cup chopped parsley
1 teaspoon black peppercorns

1) Combine olive oil, vinegar, water, garlic, oregano and salt in saucepan and bring to a boil for 5 minutes.

2) Add parsley and peppercorns. Reduce heat and simmer for about 5 minutes.

3) Add sliced mushrooms.

4) Let mushrooms marinate for about 10 minutes.

5) Drain and serve.

Snacks & Finger Foods

Raw Mushroom Surprise

1 cup small mushrooms
6 Tablespoon sour cream
3 Tablespoon milk
1/2 teaspoon lemon juice
1/2 teaspoon salt
1/2 teaspoon pepper
1 teaspoon chives

1) Wash mushrooms thoroughly and trim stems.

2) Mix sour cream, milk, lemon juice, salt and pepper in bowl.

3) Slice mushrooms paper-thin and stir into sour cream mixture.

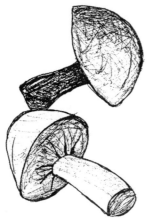

4) Stir in chives.

5) Serve with gluten-free crackers or chopped vegetables.

Snacks & Finger Foods

Beyond Rice Cakes

Stuffed Mushrooms

8 large mushrooms
6 Tablespoon sour cream
3 Tablespoon milk
1/2 teaspoon lemon juice
1/2 teaspoon salt
1/2 teaspoon pepper
1 teaspoon chives

1) Wash mushrooms and hollow out insides, discarding core.

2) Combine sour cream, milk, lemon juice, chives, salt and pepper in small bowl.

3) Spoon sour cream mixture into hollowed-out mushrooms.

Snacks & Finger Foods

Cheesy Garlic Wedges

1 loaf favorite gluten-free bread product
1 Tablespoon margarine or butter
2 Tablespoon garlic powder
1/2 cup freshly grated parmesan cheese
1/2 cup mozzarella cheese

1) Preheat oven to 350 degrees.

2) Lay gluten-free bread on foil-lined baking sheet.

3) Spread butter or margarine onto bread.

4) Sprinkle garlic powder, parmesan cheese and mozzarella cheese on top of bread.

5) Bake for 10 minutes.

6) Switch oven to broil setting, and then broil bread until cheese is golden brown.

7) Slice bread into wedges. Serve immediately.

Snacks & Finger Foods

Beyond Rice Cakes

Baked Brie & Jelly

1 wheel of favorite brand of Brie cheese
1/2 cup favorite flavor of jelly (cherry or blackberry suggested)

1) Preheat oven to 350 degrees.

2) Place Brie wheel on foil-lined baking sheet.

3) Spread jelly on top.

4) Bake for about 25 minutes.

5) Serve with favorite gluten-free crackers or bread.

Snacks & Finger Foods

Mango Salsa

* Submitted by the Palm Beach County Celiac Support Group

1 (16 oz) can black beans
1 (16 oz) can corn or 2 ears of fresh corn
1 chopped mango
1/2 chopped red pepper
1/3 cup chopped red onion
1/3 cup chopped cilantro
1/4 cup lime juice

1)   Mix all the ingredients together.

2)   Drain excess liquid.

3)   Refrigerate for 1 hour before serving.

4)   Serve as side dish with gluten-free crackers, rice cakes or as a sauce for fish, chicken etc.

Beyond Rice Cakes

Avocado & Corn Salsa

3 avocados, diced
1 tomato, diced
1 (8 oz) bag frozen corn
1/4 cup cilantro, chopped
Lime juice, to taste
Salt, to taste

1) Combine all ingredients in medium size serving bowl.

2) Serve with corn chips.

Snacks & Finger Foods

Guacamole

4 avocados
1 tomato
1 teaspoon garlic salt
1/2 cup chopped onion
1/4 cup chopped cilantro

1) Peel skin off of avocado and chop peeled avocado into small pieces.

2) Put avocado pieces into mixing bowl and mash with fork.

3) Dice tomato.

4) Chop onion into small pieces.

5) Stir tomato, onion, garlic salt and cilantro into mashed avocado.

6) Serve with corn chips.

Snacks & Finger Foods

Beyond Rice Cakes

Ants on a Log

1 bunch celery
1 cup peanut butter
1 cup raisins

1) Slice celery into 3-inch sections.

2) Spread peanut butter onto celery.

3) Top with raisins.

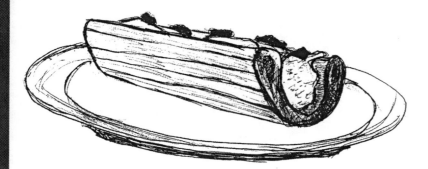

Snacks & Finger Foods

Celery & Cream Cheese

1 bunch of celery
1 cup cream cheese (your favorite flavor)
1/2 cup walnuts

1) Wash celery.

2) Slice celery into 3-inch sections.

3) Spread cream cheese onto celery.

4) Top with walnuts. Serve.

Beyond Rice Cakes

Easy Quesadillas

1 pkg corn tortillas
2 cups of your favorite cheese (cheddar and Monterey Jack work well)

**OPTIONAL: add in chicken, black beans, rice, or any other ingredients you enjoy.

1) Preheat oven or toaster oven to 300 degrees.

2) Layer cheese and add-ins between tortillas.

3) Heat using an oven or toaster oven, depending on what is available to you.

4) Bake for about 7-8 minutes.

5) Serve while hot with sour cream, guacamole and salsa.

Snacks & Finger Foods

Beyond Rice Cakes

Chewy Granola Bars

1 cup butter or margarine
3/4 cup brown sugar
1/2 cup sugar
2 Tablespoon corn syrup
4 cups buckwheat flakes
1 cup shredded coconut
1/3 cup chopped nuts
1 cup chocolate chips

1) Preheat oven to 325 degrees.

2) Grease a 12 x 9-inch cookie sheet.

3) In a large saucepan heat butter, sugars and corn syrup on low heat until melted.

4) Stir in remaining ingredients until evenly combined.

5) Spread mixture over cookie sheet and smooth surface.

6) Bake for 30 minutes.

7) Slice into bars.

Snacks & Finger Foods

Beyond Rice Cakes

Cheese Plate

1 hunk cheddar cheese
1 hunk mozzarella cheese
1 hunk Brie cheese
1 hunk Swiss cheese
1 hunk Pepper Jack cheese

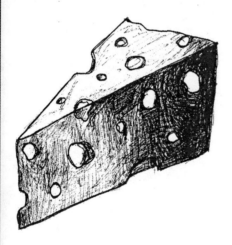

1) Slice all cheeses and arrange on platter.

2) Serve with vegetables and gluten-free crackers.

Snacks & Finger Foods

Golden Potatoes
Submitted by Danene and Abby Gooding

6 potatoes, cubed into 1-inch pieces
1 Tablespoon olive oil
1 pkg Lipton Onion Soup Mix

1) Preheat oven to 375 degrees.

2) Combine potatoes, oil and soup mix in a large bowl.

3) Pour on baking sheet and bake for 35 minutes or until potatoes are golden brown.

4) Turn over after the first 15 minutes.

5) Serve with sour cream and chives.

Beyond Rice Cakes

Popcorn Balls

4 cups marshmallows
1 cup un-popped popcorn kernels
1 cup chocolate chips
1 Tablespoon margarine
1-2 Tablespoon vegetable oil

1) In medium saucepan melt margarine and marshmallows on low heat.

2) Stir in chocolate chips.

3) In separate pot, pour oil and add popcorn on medium-high heat, stirring until popped.

4) Drizzle marshmallow mixture over popcorn and form into balls.

5) Cool on waxed paper.

6) After balls have cooled, store in airtight container.

**OPTIONAL: For an easier alternative, skip step #3 by using micro-waveable popcorn.

Snacks & Finger Foods

Connie's Famous Cornbread

1 1/4 cups all-purpose gluten-free baking flour
3/4 cup yellow corn meal
1/4 cup sugar
2 teaspoon baking powder
1/2 teaspoon salt
1 cup milk
1/4 cup vegetable oil
1 egg, beaten

1) Pre-heat oven to 400 degrees.

2) Grease an 8 or 9 inch square baking pan.

3) Combine dry ingredients.

4) With a spoon, stir in milk, oil and egg, mixing just until dry ingredients are moistened.

5) Pour batter into prepared pan.

6) Bake 20 minutes or until just light brown on the top. Serve warm with butter, cream cheese or corn syrup. Great with chili or other varieties of soup.

Snacks & Finger Foods

Beyond Rice Cakes

Banana Roll-Ups

6 bananas
1 cup peanut butter or Nutella
1/2 cup raisins
1/2 cup gluten-free granola
1/2 cup chocolate chips

1) Peel bananas and cut in half lengthwise.

2) Spread either peanut butter or Nutella all over banana pieces.

3) Combine raisins, granola and chocolate chips in bowl.

4) Sprinkle mixture on top of bananas.

5) Chill before serving. Goes great with a glass of milk.

Snacks & Finger Foods

White Bean Dip
Submitted by Mike McHenry

2 Tablespoon olive oil
1/2 medium onion, chopped
1 garlic clove, minced
1 bunch scallions, cleaned and chopped into small pieces
4 thin prosciutto slices
8 fresh basil leaves, chopped
1 15-ounce can cannellini beans, drained with liquid reserved
1 Tablespoon lemon juice
1/2 cup canned artichoke hearts, drained
Salt, to taste
Cracked black pepper, to taste

1) Add olive oil to pan and warm over medium-high heat for about 2 minutes.
2) Reduce heat to medium.
3) Add onions and garlic.
4) Sauté lightly for 2-3 minutes or until onions are translucent.
5) Add the scallions and prosciutto and simmer for about 4 minutes.
6) Remove from heat and set aside.
7) Add beans, lemon juice and the onion mixture to a food processor and process for 45-90 seconds or until thoroughly combined.
8) Add the artichoke hearts and pulse until mostly pureed with small chunks. If too thick, add the reserved cannellini bean liquid.
9) Season to taste with salt and pepper.
10) For best results, let dip sit a few hours before serving.

Snacks & Finger Foods

Simple Salads & Soups

BBQ Chicken Salad

Chunky Tuna Salad

Blackberry Spinach Salad

Watermelon & Tomato Salad

Garlic Shrimp Salad

Goat Cheese & Ham Salad

Taco Salad*

Avocado & Tomato Salad*

Curried Egg Salad

Chicken Salad*

Fresh Tuna Salad

Salmon Salad

Waldorf Salad

Potato Salad

Spinach & Walnut Salad

Grandma's Salad

Summer Salad

Veggie Pasta Salad*

Sunshine Salad

Broccoli Salad*

Chicken-Broccoli Soup

Bean-less Chili

Denotes very easy to make

BBQ Chicken Salad

1 pkg boneless skinless chicken breasts
1 (8 oz) can black beans, rinsed and dried
2 tomatoes, diced
1 avocado, chopped
1 cup chopped red or green onion
1 red, yellow, orange or green pepper, chopped
1 cup grated cheese
1 cup salsa
1/2 cup sour cream
1 head of lettuce rinsed and chopped
1/4 cup Ranch dressing
1 bag of corn chips
1 cup of your favorite BBQ sauce

1) Rinse chicken in cold water and pat dry.
2) Place in shallow glass dish or zippered storage bag.
3) Add BBQ sauce and marinate in BBQ sauce for at least one hour.
4) Grill chicken. If you do not have a grill or grill pan, place chicken on foil-lined baking sheet and cook in oven on BROIL setting for about 10 minutes on each side.
5) In large bowl, combine lettuce, black beans, tomatoes, avocado, onion, peppers, and grated cheese.
6) Toss with gluten-free ranch salad dressing.
7) Serve with salsa and sour cream on the side and garnish with corn chips.

Simple Salads & Soups

Beyond Rice Cakes

Miriam's Chunky Tuna Salad
Submitted by Miriam Berg

2 handfuls fresh spinach leaves, rinsed
1 handful grape tomatoes
2-3 sliced mushrooms
1/2 cucumber, sliced
1/2 red bell pepper, 1/2 yellow bell pepper
Handful baby carrots
1 Pink Lady apple (or your favorite sweet apple)
3 pieces of gluten-free bread
2 teaspoon olive oil
6 teaspoon balsamic vinaigrette
1/2 teaspoon basil
1 can white Albacore tuna in water

1) Mix olive oil and balsamic vinegar in small bowl or shake it up in a very small Tupperware container.
2) Slice vegetables, apple as needed. Put vegetables, apple into large bowl.
3) Open tuna can, put tuna fish on top of salad.
4) Rip up bread into little pieces and put it on top of the salad and tuna (pieces should be about 1/16 of the piece of bread)
5) Pour balsamic vinaigrette over salad, pouring more generously on the bread and tuna.
6) Sprinkle basil over salad.
7) Toss salad well. Make sure that balsamic vinaigrette seeps into bread, making it soggy.

Simple Salads & Soups

Blackberry Spinach Salad
Submitted by Amanda Klein

1 1/2 cups baby spinach
1 cup fresh blackberries
3 oz. crumbled feta
1 cup cherry tomatoes
1/2 green onion, sliced
1/4 cup Balsamic vinaigrette

1) Wash spinach and blackberries.

2) Combine spinach, feta, tomatoes and onion.

3) Toss in balsamic vinaigrette.

4) Add blackberries last.

Simple Salads & Soups

Beyond Rice Cakes

Watermelon & Tomato Salad
* Submitted by Amanda Klein

4 lbs of watermelon (preferably seedless)
2 lbs vine-ripened tomatoes (about 6 medium; preferably yellow)
1 teaspoon coarse salt (preferably sea salt)
1/2 small red onion
2 Tablespoon fresh lime juice, or to taste
1 teaspoon finely grated peeled fresh gingerroot, or to taste
1/2 teaspoon sugar

1) Remove rind and seeds from watermelon.
2) Cut fruit into 1 1/2-inch pieces and put in a large bowl.
3) Cut tomatoes into 1 1/2-inch pieces.
4) Add tomatoes and salt to watermelon, tossing to combine.
5) Let mixture stand at cool room temperature 3 hours.
6) In a colander set over a small saucepan drain mixture and transfer to a bowl. Simmer liquid until reduced to about 2 tablespoons and cool completely.
7) Halve onion and thinly slice enough to measure 1/4 cup. Add onion to watermelon mixture.
8) In a small bowl, stir together reduced watermelon-tomato juice, limejuice, gingerroot and sugar.
9) Just before serving, toss salad with juice mixture.

Simple Salads & Soups

Garlic Shrimp Salad

1 head iceberg lettuce, rinsed and chopped
1 handful fresh spinach
1 pkg baby frozen shrimp
1 tomato, diced
1 red pepper, chopped
1 red apple, diced
2 cups chopped broccoli
1 handful chopped carrots
1/4 cup goat cheese
1 Tablespoon margarine
3 teaspoon garlic powder
1 teaspoon parsley
1/4 cup gluten-free balsamic vinaigrette salad dressing

1) Defrost shrimp and sauté in skillet with margarine, garlic powder and parsley until shrimp turn pink.

2) In separate bowl combine lettuce, spinach, tomato, peppers, apple, broccoli and carrots.

3) Toss in shrimp and goat cheese.

4) Mix in gluten-free balsamic vinaigrette salad dressing.

5) Serve immediately.

Simple Salads & Soups

Beyond Rice Cakes

Goat Cheese & Ham Salad

1 head iceberg lettuce, rinsed and chopped
1 handful fresh spinach, rinsed
1 pkg pre-cooked ham
1 lbs mushrooms, sliced
1 tomato diced
1 red pepper, chopped
1 red apple, diced
2 cups broccoli, chopped
1 handful carrots, chopped
1/2 cup goat cheese
1 Tablespoon margarine
1/4 cup gluten-free honey mustard salad dressing

1) Melt margarine in skillet on medium heat.

2) Add ham and mushrooms, cooking until ham browns, about 5-7 minutes. Set aside.

3) In a large salad bowl combine lettuce, spinach, tomato, red pepper, broccoli and carrots.

4) Gently mix in ham and mushrooms.

5) Sprinkle goat cheese on top.

6) Serve chilled with gluten-free honey mustard salad dressing.

Simple Salads & Soups

Taco Salad

1 lb ground beef
3 teaspoon garlic powder
3 teaspoon onion powder
1 (8 oz) can black beans or refried beans
2 tomatoes, diced
1 avocado, chopped (can substitute guacamole)
1 cup chopped red or green onion
1 red, yellow, orange or green pepper, chopped
1 cup grated cheddar cheese
1 cup salsa
1/2 cup sour cream
1 head lettuce
1 bag of corn chips

1) Brown ground beef in skillet, draining grease after beef is cooked.
2) Season beef with garlic powder and onion powder.
3) Line platter with corn chips.
4) Warm beans for about 45 seconds in small microwave-safe bowl and then spread on top of corn chips.
5) Layer ground beef on top of beans.
6) In separate bowl toss together tomatoes, avocado, onion, peppers and lettuce. Add on top of beans and meat.
7) Sprinkle grated cheddar cheese on top and garnish with salsa and sour cream.
8) Serve immediately.

Simple Salads & Soups

Beyond Rice Cakes

Avocado & Tomato Salad

3 avocados
2 tomatoes
1/2 large onion
1/2 cup cilantro
1 finely chopped jalapeno pepper
4 Tablespoon lime juice
2 teaspoon salt, to taste
2 teaspoon pepper, to taste

1) Chop avocados into 1/2-inch pieces.

2) Dice tomatoes and onion.

3) Mix avocados, tomatoes and onions in large salad bowl with cilantro and jalapeno peppers.

4) Add lime juice, salt and pepper to taste.

5) Serve with corn chips.

Simple Salads & Soups

Curried Egg Salad
Submitted by Amanda Klein

1/3 cup mayonnaise
1 Tablespoon fresh lime juice
1 1/2 teaspoon curry powder
1 teaspoon Dijon mustard
1/4 teaspoon salt
1/8 teaspoon cayenne pepper
6 large hard-boiled large eggs, chopped
1 cup diced red apple
1/3 cup finely chopped red onion
1/4 cup chopped cilantro

1) Whisk together mayonnaise, lime juice, curry powder, mustard, salt and cayenne in a bowl until mixture is smooth.

2) Add chopped eggs, apple, onion and cilantro.

3) Stir all together.

4) Serve with gluten-free crackers.

Beyond Rice Cakes

Chicken Salad

4 boneless skinless chicken breasts
1 bunch celery, rinsed
1/2 cup dried cranberries
1/4 cup mayonnaise
1 teaspoon paprika
1 dash salt
1 dash pepper

1) Rinse chicken and pat dry.

2) Preheat oven to 350 degrees.

3) Season chicken with salt, pepper and paprika.

4) Bake chicken for about 45 minutes or until fully cooked.

5) Allow to cool.

6) Chop chicken into small cubes.

7) Chop celery into small pieces.

8) Stir chicken, celery, cranberries and mayonnaise together in salad bowl.

9) Serve with favorite gluten-free bread or with chips.

Simple Salads & Soups

Fresh Tuna Salad

1 or 2 pieces fresh tuna (Ahi)
1 dash pepper
1 dash salt
1 Tablespoon lemon juice
1 head lettuce, rinsed and chopped
1 tomato
1 avocado
2 Tablespoon gluten-free Asian vinaigrette salad dressing (balsamic vinaigrette works well too)

1) Preheat oven on BROIL setting.

2) Season tuna with pepper, salt and lemon juice.

3) Allow tuna to broil until cooked about halfway through (about 6-7 minutes).

4) Slice tuna into long strips.

5) Toss lettuce, tomato, avocado and salad dressing together in salad bowl.

6) Arrange greens on plates.

7) Top with hot sliced tuna.

8) Serve immediately.

Simple Salads & Soups

Beyond Rice Cakes

Salmon Salad

1 piece of fresh salmon steak for every person eating
1 Tablespoon lemon juice per piece of salmon
1 dash salt
1 dash peppercorn seasoning
1 head lettuce, rinsed and chopped.
1 tomato
2 Tablespoon gluten-free balsamic vinaigrette salad dressing

1) Preheat oven on BROIL setting.

2) Season fresh salmon steaks with lemon juice, salt and peppercorn seasoning.

3) Broil salmon about 5 minutes then flip over and cook another 5 minutes.

4) In salad bowl combine chopped lettuce, tomato and gluten-free balsamic vinaigrette salad dressing.

5) Place salmon on top of greens.

6) Serve immediately.

Simple Salads & Soups

Waldorf Salad

2 red apples diced (remove core but do not peel)
2 stalks celery diced
1 cup seedless grapes cut in half
1/4 cup raisins
1/3 cup walnuts chopped
1/4 cup mayonnaise
1 teaspoon sugar
1 dash salt

1) Dice apples and celery and cut seedless grapes in half.

2) Combine apples, celery, grapes, raisins and walnuts.

3) Add mayonnaise, sugar and salt.

4) Stir well. Serve chilled.

**OPTIONAL: before serving add favorite grated cheese to top.

Simple Salads & Soups

Beyond Rice Cakes

Potato Salad

4 large russet baking potatoes, scrubbed and quartered
1 green onion chopped
1 bunch celery chopped
2 hardboiled eggs
1 Tablespoon pickled relish
1/4 teaspoon yellow mustard
1/4 cup mayonnaise (enough to make moist)
Salt to taste
Pepper to taste
Onion powder to taste

1) In large pot, boil water.

2) Add potatoes and allow to cook for about 30 minutes.

3) Peel partially, leaving some skin on potatoes.

4) Cut potatoes into ½-inch cubes.

5) Chop green onion, celery and hardboiled eggs.

6) Mix potatoes, onion, celery, egg, relish, mustard and mayonnaise together.

7) Add salt and pepper to taste.

Simple Salads & Soups

Spinach & Walnut Salad

1 pkg fresh spinach, rinsed and drained
1 cup dried cranberries
1 cup walnuts
1/4 cup gluten-free Italian salad dressing

1) Toss spinach, cranberries and walnuts together.

2) Drizzle dressing over salad and toss together.

3) Serve as a side salad.

Simple Salads & Soups

Beyond Rice Cakes

Grandma's Favorite Salad
*In loving memory of Lela Mae Beach

1 (12 oz) carton cottage cheese

1 (9 oz) can crushed pineapple

1 cup grated carrots

1 cup miniature marshmallows

1 Tablespoon lemon juice

1/2 teaspoon salt

2 Tablespoon sugar

1/2 cup favorite gluten-free salad dressing

1 head iceberg lettuce

1) Combine cottage cheese, pineapple, grated carrots, marshmallows, salad dressing, lemon juice, sugar and salt.

2) Chill for about 2 hours.

3) Serve in chilled lettuce cups.

Simple Salads & Soups

Summer Salad

1 head fresh broccoli
1 head fresh cauliflower
1 tomato
1 avocado
1 cucumber
1 red onion
1 red cabbage
1/2 cup raisins
1/2 cup sunflower seeds
1/4 cup gluten-free bleu cheese salad dressing

1) Chop all vegetables.

2) Toss together with raisins and sunflower seeds.

3) Drizzle bleu cheese salad dressing over mixture, then toss.

Simple Salads & Soups

Beyond Rice Cakes

Veggie Pasta Salad

1 pkg gluten-free elbow noodles
1 tomato
1 zucchini
1 red onion
1 avocado
1 lbs mushrooms
1 head broccoli
1/2 lbs carrots
1/2 cup gluten-free Italian salad dressing

1) Cook noodles in boiling salted water.

2) Drain and cool in large bowl.

3) Chop all vegetables, then stir into bowl with noodles.

4) Stir in gluten-free Italian salad dressing (enough to moisten).

5) Serve with fresh pepper.

Simple Salads & Soups

Sunshine Salad

1 (3oz) package lemon Jello
1 cup hot water
1 cup pineapple syrup
2 1/2 cup crushed pineapple drained
1 Tablespoon vinegar
1/4 teaspoon salt
1 cup grated carrots

1) Dissolve Jello in hot water.

2) Add pineapple syrup, vinegar and salt.

3) Chill until Jello is slightly thickened.

4) Fold in pineapple and carrots.

5) Serve with chopped nuts if desired.

Simple Salads & Soups

Beyond Rice Cakes

Broccoli Salad

2 cups broccoli tops
2 cups cauliflower
1/4 cup red onion, chopped
1/2 cup celery, chopped
1/2 cucumber, chopped
1/4 cup raisins
1/2 cup bacon bits
3/4 cup sour cream
2/3 cup mayonnaise
3 Tablespoon sugar

1) Chop all vegetables and mix together with raisins and bacon bits.

2) In separate bowl, combine sour cream, mayonnaise and sugar for dressing.

3) Mix all together.

Simple Salads & Soups

Chicken-Broccoli Soup

1/2 cup sweet onion, chopped
1/2 + 1 1/4 cup water
1 cup cooked chicken, diced
1 cup broccoli florets
1 cup heavy cream
1 3/4 cup cheddar cheese, shredded
Pepper, to taste
Salt, to taste

1)   In large saucepan brown onions and 1/2 cup water.

2)   Add chicken, cream, broccoli, pepper and 1 1/4 cup water.

3)   Slowly add cheese, stirring constantly.

4)   Add salt and pepper to taste.

Simple Salads & Soups

Beyond Rice Cakes

Bean-less Chili

2 pounds ground beef (lean)
1 sweet onion, chopped
4 teaspoon chili powder
1 garlic clove, minced
1/2 teaspoon crushed oregano
2 (16oz) cans tomatoes, diced with liquid
Salt, to taste
Pepper, to taste

1) In large pot, brown ground beef and onions.

2) Stir in all remaining ingredients.

3) Allow to simmer for about 2 1/2 hours.

Simple Salads & Soups

Main Dishes & Vegetables

Eggplant Pizza*
Crustless Spinach Quiche
Lettuce Roll-Ups*
Meat & Cheese Roll-Ups*
Crunchy Pepper & Tuna Salad*
Crunchy Pepper & Chicken Salad*
Risotto
Easy Enchiladas
Italian Chicken Cutlets
Salmon & Herb Rub
Roast Chicken
Polenta
Polenta Lasagna
Tamale Pie*
Ground Turkey Casserole*
Chicken & Green Pepper Casserole*
Veggie Casserole
Chopped Chicken Liver
Ground Beef & Spinach Casserole
Sour Cream Supreme
Meatless Moussaka
Baked Ziti
Ham & Swiss Pie

Cheeseburger Pie
Chicken Wings
Grilled Tomatoes*
Baked Potato*
Baked Sweet Potato*
Oven Roasted Potatoes*
Whipped Sweet Potato Bake
Indian Corn Pudding
Baked Chicken Pasta Salad*
Rice Pilaf
Tortilla Lasagna
Noodle Kugel
Hush Puppies
Swiss Vegetable Medley*
Green Bean Casserole*
Tomato & Rice Soup
Cheesy Cauliflower
Crustless Broccoli & Ham Quiche
Chicken Parmesan
Homemade Macaroni & Cheese
Lemon-Soaked Broccoli
Sautéed Spinach
Lemony Endive Salad

Denotes very easy to make

98

Beyond Rice Cakes

Eggplant Pizza
Submitted by Lianne Woolley

1 large eggplant
1 cup of tomato pasta sauce
1 cup of shredded mozzarella cheese
Salt, to taste
Pepper, to taste
Oregano, to taste
Garlic powder, to taste

1) Preheat oven to 350 degrees.

2) Slice the eggplant lengthwise into 1/2-inch thick slices and lay on a greased backing tray.

3) Cover each slice to the edges with sauce.

4) Add seasoning to taste.

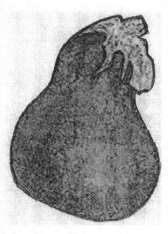

5) Top with mozzarella.

6) Cook for 10 to 15 minutes or until cheese browns.

**OPTIONAL: Add more vegetables (onions, peppers, mushrooms, fresh tomatoes, roasted red peppers) to vary the taste. To ensure that the veggies stick to the pizza, add a thin layer of cheese on top to secure them.

Main Dishes & Vegetables

Crustless Spinach Quiche
Submitted by Amanda Klein

1 Tablespoon vegetable oil or cooking spray
1 onion, chopped
1 (10 oz) pkg frozen chopped spinach, thawed and drained
5 eggs, beaten
3 cups shredded Muenster cheese (or your favorite type of cheese)
1/4 teaspoon salt
1/8 teaspoon ground black pepper
Optional: ham, tomatoes, mushrooms, whatever you'd like!

1) Preheat oven to 350 degrees.
2) Lightly grease a 9-inch pie pan.
3) Heat oil in a large skillet over medium-high heat.

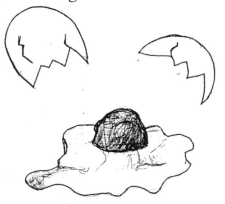

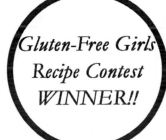

Gluten-Free Girls
Recipe Contest
WINNER!!

4) Add onions and cook, stiring occasionally, until onions are soft. Stir in spinach and other mix-ins and continue cooking until excess moisture has evaporated.
5) In a large bowl combine eggs, cheese, salt and pepper. Add spinach mixture and stir to blend.
6) Scoop into prepared pie pan.
7) Bake in preheated oven until eggs have set, about 30 minutes.
8) Let cool for 10 minutes before serving.

Main Dishes & Vegetables

Beyond Rice Cakes

Lettuce Roll-Ups
*Submitted by Lianne Woolley

4-6 large iceberg lettuce leaves (washed and dried)
2 Tablespoon cream cheese (softened)
1 Tablespoon hot sauce
3 oz sliced deli turkey
1 finely sliced or chopped tomato
Salt, to taste
Pepper, to taste

1) In a small bowl, combine the cream cheese with the hot sauce to form a smooth, pale brown mixture.

2) Lay lettuce leaves on a large plate and spread a 1/4-inch layer of the cream cheese mixture on top of one side of them.

3) Add a few layers of turkey, then the tomatoes, then another few layers of turkey (it sticks better this way).

4) Add salt and pepper to taste.

5) Roll the lettuce leaves from tip to stem to make a tube shape.

6) Cut and serve.

Main Dishes & Vegetables

Meat & Cheese Roll-Ups

1 lbs deli meat (turkey, roast beef, ham, pastrami)
1 lbs sliced cheese (Swiss, cheddar, Monterey Jack, havarti, muenster)
1 teaspoon honey mustard
1 teaspoon mayonnaise
Sliced tomato
Leaf lettuce

1) Lay slices of cheese flat on a plate.

2) Spread mayonnaise and mustard onto cheese.

3) Layer with favorite deli meat, tomato and lettuce.

4) Serve with chips.

Main Dishes & Vegetables

Beyond Rice Cakes

Crunchy Pepper & Tuna Salad

1 can Albacore tuna in water
1 Tablespoon pickled relish
1 hard-boiled egg
1 Tablespoon mayonnaise
Dash of mustard
1 pepper (red, green, orange or yellow)

1) In bowl mash tuna, relish, hard-boiled egg, mayonnaise and mustard together.

2) Slice pepper in half and remove seeds.

3) Spoon tuna salad into pepper halves.

4) Serve with chips.

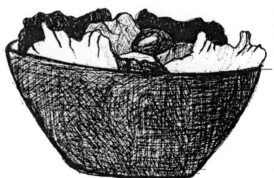

Main Dishes & Vegetables

Crunchy Pepper & Chicken Salad

2 boneless skinless chicken breasts (about 1 lb)
1 bunch celery, rinsed
1/2 cup dried cranberries
1/4 cup mayonnaise
1 teaspoon paprika
1 dash salt
1 dash pepper
1 pepper (red, green, orange or yellow)

1) Preheat oven to 350 degrees.
2) Rinse chicken and pat dry.
3) Season chicken with salt, pepper and paprika.
4) Bake chicken for about 45 minutes or until fully cooked.
5) Allow to cool. Chop chicken into small cubes.
6) Chop celery into small pieces.
7) Stir chicken, celery, cranberries and mayonnaise together in salad bowl.
8) Slice pepper in half and remove seeds.
9) Spoon chicken salad into pepper halves.
10) Serve with chips.

Main Dishes & Vegetables

Beyond Rice Cakes

Risotto

1 cup risotto Italian style rice
2 Tablespoon olive oil
1/2 cup chopped onion
1/2 cup sliced mushrooms
3 cups (approximately) of chicken or vegetable broth
1 pkg frozen chopped spinach, thawed
1/4 cup grated freshly grated parmesan cheese

1) Place onion, mushrooms, and olive oil in a saucepan.
2) Sauté on medium heat until onion is clear.
3) Add the rice and sauté, stirring until all grains are coated with oil, and the rice starts to turn golden, about 2 minutes.
4) Add 1 cup of the broth. Stir until liquid is absorbed.
5) Gradually stir remaining broth 1 cup at a time, cooking and stirring until liquid is absorbed before adding the next cup. When rice is almost soft, add the chopped spinach and freshly grated parmesan cheese.
6) Stir a few minutes longer, then turn out into a serving bowl.
7) Top with extra parmesan cheese. Good as a side dish, or as a vegetarian main dish served with a salad.

<u>Microwave instructions.</u>

Combine 1 cup rice, 2 Tablespoon butter or oil, and 3 cups warm broth in a microwave-safe round casserole. Cover; microwave on high about 18 minutes. Stir 2 or 3 times during process. Add drained, thawed chopped spinach and freshly grated parmesan cheese. Remove from microwave, stir. Let stand covered 5 minutes.

Main Dishes & Vegetables

Easy Enchiladas

1 pkg corn tortillas
1 pkg grated cheese (blend of cheddar and mozzarella works well)

For Sauce:
2 cups tomato sauce
3 cups water
1/2 teaspoon onion powder
1/4 teaspoon garlic powder
3 Tablespoon chili powder
4 Tablespoon cornstarch

1) In a saucepan, combine all SAUCE ingredients. Stir constantly and cook over medium heat until mixture comes to a boil.
2) Reduce heat to medium and allow to simmer about five minutes until mixture thickens.
3) Set aside.
4) Preheat oven to 350 degrees.
5) Line casserole dish with thin layer of sauce.
6) Fill each corn tortilla with handful of cheese and roll.
7) Layer in casserole dish and top with sauce.
8) Sprinkle cheese on top of tortilla rolls and bake for 25 minutes.
9) Serve with guacamole, sour cream and corn chips.

Main Dishes & Vegetables

Beyond Rice Cakes

A more difficult alternative...
Sour Cream Enchiladas
*Submitted by Karina Allrich

<u>Filling:</u>
2 cups cooked, torn or shredded chicken pieces
1 cup sour cream (dairy-free alternative: gluten-free mayonnaise)
Fresh lime juice from 1 lime
Lemon pepper seasoning, to taste
1/4 teaspoon ground cumin

<u>Sauce:</u>
2 (4 oz) cans chopped green chilies
1 (16 oz) jar of your favorite green or red salsa, or tomato sauce

To Assemble Shell:
10 white or yellow corn tortillas
2 cups shredded Monterey Jack, Colby, or cheddar cheese

1) Preheat oven to 350 degrees. Lightly oil a 13 x 9 x 2-inch baking dish.

2) In a mixing bowl toss together the cooked chicken, sour cream, lime juice and seasonings.

Continued...

Main Dishes & Vegetables

3) In a large measuring cup (or bowl), combine the green chilies, with the salsa or tomato sauce; spread 1/4 cup of this sauce in the bottom of the oiled baking dish.

4) Heat the tortillas by wrapping them in a clean paper towel and microwaving them for less than one minute; or, if you prefer, heat the tortillas individually one by one in a non-stick skillet until softened.

5) To fill the tortillas, lay one tortilla in the prepared baking dish, wetting it with the sauce.

6) Spoon a generous tablespoon of the chicken mixture down the center of the tortilla and roll it up into place, seam side down. Repeat for the remaining tortillas.

7) Spoon the sauce all over the rolled tortillas and top with shredded cheese.

8) Bake for 20 minutes (or until the cheese is melted and the enchiladas are hot).

9) Serve with sour cream, guacamole and salsa

Main Dishes & Vegetables

Beyond Rice Cakes

Italian Chicken Cutlets
*Submitted by Elaine R. Grabar

2 lbs thinly cut chicken breasts
2 Tablespoon extra-virgin olive oil
1 1/2 cups of your favorite gluten-free flour
2 Tablespoon potato starch flour
1 Tablespoon corn starch
2 eggs beaten (alternative: 3 egg whites)
2 teaspoon Italian spices (salt, onion powder, garlic powder, dried basil, & dried oregano)
3 cloves of fresh garlic
Sprinkle of chili powder
1/2 cup of freshly grated Parmesan cheese

1) Wash the chicken under cold water and pat dry.
2) Cut the breasts into thin large-size cutlets.
3) Marinade the chicken in extra-virgin olive oil, fresh garlic, and salt for a minimum of one hour.
4) Dip the chicken into a mixture of beaten egg and some of the Italian spices. Then, dip the chicken into mixture of gluten-free flour, potato starch flour, cornstarch, remaining spices, chili powder, and freshly grated parmesan cheese.
5) Cook the coated chicken cutlets, using a non-stick skillet, in pre-heated olive oil or your favorite healthy cooking oil on medium-high heat, until each side is golden brown. This usually takes about 6 minutes on each side.
6) Place cooked chicken cutlets on paper towels to absorb extra oil.
7) Enjoy with your favorite vegetables!!

Main Dishes & Vegetables

Salmon & Herb Rub
Submitted by Amanda Klein

1/4 cup fresh cilantro or parsley, chopped very fine (or 1 teaspoon dried)
1/4 cup fresh dill, chopped very fine (or 1 teaspoon dried)
1 teaspoon black pepper
1 Tablespoon plus 1 teaspoon olive oil
Salmon steaks, about 1" thick (enough for everyone eating)
Vegetable cooking spray

1) Combine cilantro, dill, pepper and olive oil in small bowl; stir together to combine.

2) Rinse salmon and pat dry.

3) Place in shallow pan; spread herb rub evenly on both sides of salmon steaks.

4) Cover and marinate in refrigerator for 20 minutes.

5) Preheat grill or broiler.

6) Place salmon on grill rack or broiler pan coated with cooking spray.

7) Grill 5 to 7 minutes on each side or until salmon is done and flakes to fork. If using a broiler, cook each side for about 4 minutes.

Main Dishes & Vegetables

Beyond Rice Cakes

Roast Chicken
Submitted by Amanda Klein

1 (3.5 to 4 lb) whole chicken, rinsed and patted dry
1 1/2 Tablespoon salt
2 teaspoons cracked white pepper
1 lemon, halved
2 fresh bay leaves
6 cloves garlic, roughly chopped
4 sprigs rosemary, roughly chopped, plus 1 tablespoon for gravy
2 Tablespoon olive oil
2 Tablespoon unsalted butter, at room temperature
1 cup chicken stock
2 Tablespoon roasted garlic
1 cup dry white wine

1) Preheat the oven to 450 degrees.

2) In a 9 x 13-inch roasting pan, add the carrots, celery and onions. Season the chicken both inside and out with the kosher salt and white pepper.

3) Squeeze the lemon halves over the chicken and place the rinds inside the cavity. Place the bay leaves inside the cavity.

Continued…

Main Dishes & Vegetables

4)   In a small bowl, combine the garlic, rosemary, olive oil and butter. Rub the chicken both inside and out with the garlic rosemary blend and place in the roasting pan.

5)   Place the pan in the oven and roast the chicken for 40 to 50 minutes, or until the juices run clear. To test this, insert a thermometer in the thickest part of a leg. It should register at 160 degrees internal temperature.

6)   Remove the chicken from the oven and allow to cool for 10 to 15 minutes before carving. Pour off excess fat from pan and return to heat.

7)   Whisk in chicken stock, roasted garlic, white wine and chopped rosemary, scraping up the bits on the bottom of pan. Bring to a boil, and then reduce to a simmer. Reduce gravy by half, until thickened. Serve chicken with gravy on the side.

Beyond Rice Cakes

Polenta

4 cups water
1 cup corn meal
1 teaspoon salt
1/4 cup grated freshly grated parmesan cheese

1) Bring the water to a boil.

2) Slowly pour in the corn meal and salt, stirring constantly.

3) Cook until thickened, about 10 minutes, or until the polenta starts to pull away from the sides of the pan.

4) Stir in the freshly grated parmesan cheese.

5) Pour into a square or loaf pan. It will be like mush when hot, but after cooling, it will set, and you can slice it.

6) Serve warm with milk or margarine.

**OPTIONAL: This is also good topped with a marinara sauce. Heat the sauce in the microwave or on the stove top. Pour over the polenta and top with freshly grated parmesan cheese or grated mozzarella cheese.

Main Dishes & Vegetables

Polenta Lasagna
Submitted by Karina Allrich

2 rolls of pre-cooked polenta, drained
2 Tablespoon olive oil
2-3 cups assorted sliced veggies: peppers, onions, mushrooms, broccoli, etc.
1 teaspoon Italian herb seasoning
1 teaspoon dried basil
2 cloves garlic, minced (or use garlic powder)
3 cups marinara sauce
1 cup shredded mozzarella cheese or 1 (4 oz) block Feta cheese, crumbled
1/2 cup sliced olives, black or green
Grated freshly grated parmesan

1) Preheat oven to 350 degrees.
2) Spray or lightly oil a 13 x 9 lasagna-style baking dish.
3) Heat olive oil in a skillet and sauté the vegetables until they are tender-crisp. Season with Italian herbs, basil and garlic.
4) Stir for one minute; remove from heat. Set aside.
5) Using a sharp knife, carefully slice the polenta lengthwise into long thin strips, or cut round slices crosswise.
6) Spoon 1/4 cup of pasta sauce into the oiled baking dish and spread around bottom of dish. Make a layer with half of the polenta slices, followed by a layer of half of the veggies, then half the jar of red sauce.
7) Add half the cheese. Make another layer of polenta, veggies, and red sauce.
8) Top it off with the remaining cheese. Stud the top with sliced olives and extra cheese, if desired.
9) Sprinkle on more Italian herbs and basil.
10) Bake 20 minutes or until hot and bubbly.

Main Dishes & Vegetables

Beyond Rice Cakes

Tamale Pie

2 cans chili (one with beans, one without beans)
2 cans creamed corn
1 can sliced black olives
6 tamales (make sure they are gluten-free)
3 cups shredded cheddar and mozzarella cheese (a mixed variety)
Sour cream
Guacamole
Salsa
Corn chips

1) Preheat oven to 350 degrees.

2) Mix all ingredients together in large bowl.

3) Pour into large casserole dish or pie tin.

4) Top with grated cheese.

5) Bake for 45 minutes.

6) Serve with sour cream, guacamole, salsa and corn chips.

Main Dishes & Vegetables

Ground Turkey Casserole

1 lb ground turkey
1/2 lb fresh mushrooms
1 cup onion
1 pkg frozen spinach
2 (8 oz) cans gluten-free tomato soup
2 (8 oz) cans gluten-free cream of mushroom soup
1 pkg gluten-free pasta
2 cups grated mozzarella cheese
1 Tablespoon ketchup
Salt to taste
Pepper to taste

1) Preheat oven to 350 degrees.
2) In large skillet brown turkey, onions, spinach and mushrooms. Season with ketchup, salt and pepper.
3) In large pot boil water. Add pasta and cook until tender.
4) Drain pasta and put back in large pot.
5) Combine meat mixture with pasta and pour in 1 can of tomato soup and 1 can of cream of mushroom soup.
6) Stir in one cup mozzarella cheese.
7) Stir all together. Pour into large casserole dish.
8) Evenly pour remaining tomato soup and cream of mushroom soup over top.
9) Sprinkle remaining mozzarella cheese on top.
10) Bake 35-40 minutes.
11) Serve immediately.

Main Dishes & Vegetables

Beyond Rice Cakes

Chicken & Green Pepper Casserole

4 boneless skinless chicken breasts
4 green peppers diced
1 onion, chopped
2 (8 oz) cans gluten-free cream of mushroom soup
1 pkg gluten-free pasta
1 cup freshly grated parmesan cheese
Salt, to taste
Pepper, to taste

1) Rinse chicken and pat dry.
2) Preheat oven to 350 degrees.
3) Dice chicken into 1-inch cubes and sauté with chopped onion and green peppers. Season with salt and pepper.
4) In large pot boil water.
5) Add pasta and cook until tender.
6) Drain and put back in pot.
7) Combine chicken mixture with pasta and stir in cream of mushroom soup.
8) Pour into large casserole dish.
9) Sprinkle freshly grated parmesan cheese on top.
10) Bake for 30 to 35 minutes.
11) Serve immediately.

Main Dishes & Vegetables

Veggie Casserole

1 green pepper
1 red pepper
1 yellow pepper
1 onion
1 head of broccoli
1 cup chopped carrots
1 cup gluten-free cream of mushroom soup
1/4 cup milk
1 pkg gluten-free pasta
1 cup freshly grated parmesan cheese
Salt to taste
Pepper to taste
Italian herb seasoning

1) Preheat oven to 350 degrees.
2) Chop all vegetables.
3) In large skillet sauté until veggies are tender. Season with salt, pepper and Italian herb seasoning.
4) In large pot boil water.
5) Add pasta and cook until tender. Drain and put back in pot.
6) Stir vegetables, cream of mushroom soup and milk together.
7) Pour into casserole dish. Sprinkle freshly grated parmesan cheese on top.
8) Bake for 30 to 35 minutes.

Main Dishes & Vegetables

Beyond Rice Cakes

Chopped Chicken Liver
Submitted by Sophie Silver

1 lbs fresh chicken livers
1 large or 2 small onions
4 eggs
3 Tablespoon canola or vegetable oil
Salt and pepper, to taste

1) Hard boil eggs and set aside.

2) Dice onions and set aside 2 Tablespoon.

3) Fry the rest of the diced onions in frying pan with oil.

4) When the onions are translucent, add chicken livers into the frying pan and season with salt and pepper until livers are cooked and appear brown.

5) Mash hard boiled eggs, liver, cooked onion, and liquid from onions and liver pan together using a hand blender, or large fork, if no hand blender is available.

6) Garnish with raw onions and serve.

Main Dishes & Vegetables

Ground Beef & Spinach Casserole

2 lbs ground beef
1/4 lb sliced mushrooms
1 chopped onion
1/4 cup chopped celery
1 crushed clove of garlic
1 (8 oz) pkg gluten-free macaroni pasta
1 pkg chopped spinach
1/2 cup shredded Swiss cheese
3/4 cup milk
3/4 teaspoon salt
1/4 teaspoon pepper

1) Preheat oven to 350 degrees.

2) Combine beef, onion, celery, mushrooms and garlic in large skillet until meat is brown and vegetables are tender.

3) Add spices while sautéing.

4) Combine with cooked noodles, milk and cheese.

5) Pour into casserole dish.

6) Sprinkle Swiss cheese on top.

7) Bake for 30 minutes or until top looks crunchy.

Main Dishes & Vegetables

Beyond Rice Cakes

Sour Cream Supreme

3 lbs ground beef
2 cloves minced garlic
2 (8 oz) cans tomato sauce
1 teaspoon sugar
1 teaspoon salt
1 teaspoon pepper
2 1/2 cups gluten-free elbow noodles
1 cup sour cream
1 (3 oz) pkg cream cheese
5 green onions, chopped
1 cup grated Monterey Jack and cheddar cheese

1) Preheat oven to 350 degrees.
2) Brown meat and garlic; drain off excess fat.
3) Add tomato sauce, sugar, salt and pepper. Reduce heat. Allow to simmer for 15 minutes.
4) Boil water in separate pot. Add gluten-free pasta. Cook until tender. Drain pasta.
5) Pour pasta back in to large pot.
6) In small bowl, combine sour cream, cream cheese and green onions.
7) Layer bottom of casserole dish with gluten-free noodles.
8) Pour meat sauce over top of noodles.
9) Pour sour cream and cream cheese mixture over top and bake.
10) Top with grated cheese.
11) Bake for 30 minutes.

Main Dishes & Vegetables

Meatless Moussaka

1 eggplant
2 medium zucchinis
8 oz firm tofu
1/4 cup fresh basil
2 Tablespoon chopped parsley
1 (26 oz) jar marinara sauce
2 Tablespoon freshly grated parmesan cheese
1/4 cup grated cheddar and mozzarella cheese mixed

1) Preheat oven to 350 degrees.
2) Cut eggplant crosswise into 1/2 inch thick pieces.
3) Cut zucchini into thick slices.
4) Crumble tofu in separate bowl.
5) Layer eggplant and zucchini in the bottom of 11x7-inch baking dish.
6) Sprinkle tofu over the vegetables. Top with basil and parsley.
7) Pour marinara sauce over all.
8) Bake for 30 minutes, then sprinkle with grated cheddar and mozzarella cheeses.
9) Cook for another 10 minutes or until bubbly and vegetables are tender.

**OPTIONAL: For non-vegetarian Moussaka, consider substituting ground lamb or ground beef in place of tofu.

Main Dishes & Vegetables

Beyond Rice Cakes

Danny's Baked Ziti
Submitted by Danny Tobias

1 pkg gluten-free ziti-shaped pasta (rice noodles work best)
1 (26 oz) jar spaghetti sauce
1 (15 oz) container ricotta cheese
1 (8 oz) pkg shredded mozzarella cheese, divided
1/4 cup grated freshly grated parmesan cheese

1) Preheat oven to 350 degrees.

2) Cook pasta as directed on package.

3) Drain pasta, reserving 1/2 cup of the pasta cooking water.

4) Mix spaghetti sauce, ricotta cheese and reserved pasta cooking water in large bowl.

5) Add pasta and 1/2 cup of the mozzarella cheese. Mix lightly.

6) Spoon into 13 x 9 inch baking dish sprayed with cooking spray

7) Sprinkle with remaining mozzarella cheese and the freshly grated parmesan cheese.

8) Cover with foil. Bake for 30 minutes.

9) Uncover and bake an additional 10 minute or until heated through.

Main Dishes & Vegetables

Ham & Swiss Pie

2 cups chopped ham
1 cup shredded Swiss cheese
1/3 cup green onion chopped
4 eggs
2 cups milk
1/4 teaspoon salt
1/8 teaspoon pepper

1) Preheat oven to 400 degrees.

2) Grease pie plate.

3) In skillet brown ham.

4) Sprinkle ham, cheese and onions onto pie plate.

5) Beat remaining ingredients until smooth.

6) Pour into pie plate on top of ham mixture.

7) Bake until top is golden brown and knife inserted in center comes out clean (35 to 40 minutes).

8) Cool 5 minutes before serving.

9) Serve with green salad or fresh fruit.

Main Dishes & Vegetables

Cheeseburger Pie

1 lb ground beef or turkey
1 cup chopped onion
1/2 teaspoon salt
1 cup shredded cheddar cheese
1 cup milk
1/2 cup gluten-free flour
2 eggs

1) Preheat oven to 400 degrees.

2) Grease 9-inch pie plate.

3) Brown ground beef and onion. Add in salt.

4) Pour into pie plate and sprinkle cheese on top.

5) In separate bowl, mix together milk, eggs and gluten-free flour.

6) Pour on top of beef and cheese.

7) Bake 25 to 30 minutes.

Main Dishes & Vegetables

Chicken Wings

15-20 chicken wings, tips removed and parts separated
2 cups cornstarch
4 Tablespoon oil (enough to form thin layer in bottom of frying pan)
Organic Tamari wheat-free soy sauce

1) Season wings with salt, pepper and garlic powder.

2) Place in a large bowl.

3) Pour gluten-free soy sauce over the wings so they are just barely covered. Let marinate for about 30 minutes.

4) Place cornstarch in a Ziplock-type bag.

5) Add the wings about three at a time and shake to cover with the cornstarch. Continue with the rest of the wings.

6) Place wings in a pan of hot oil and fry until golden brown, about 15 to 20 minutes, turning often.

7) Place on a platter and enjoy!!

Main Dishes & Vegetables

Beyond Rice Cakes

Grilled Tomatoes
Submitted by Amanda Klein

2 large (beafsteak size) red tomatoes
Olive oil
Salt, to taste
Pepper, to taste
Fresh basil, to taste

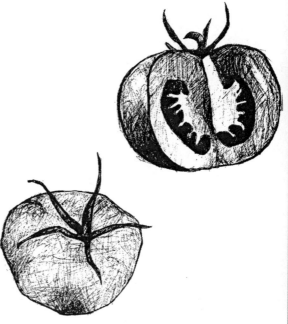

1) Slice tomatoes in half.
2) Coat top and bottom generously with olive oil.
3) Sprinkle salt and pepper on top of tomato halves as desired.
4) Top with basil.
5) Place topside down on grill or broiler (Foreman Grill also works well).
6) After 5 minutes, turn over.
7) Grill another 5 minutes or until the tomatoes start to brown at the edges and get soft.
8) Serve immediately.

Main Dishes & Vegetables

Baked Potato

1 large baking potato (washed well)
1/2 cup frozen broccoli (or other favorite vegetable)
1/4 cup shredded cheddar cheese

1) Poke 2 holes in the potato with a knife so it won't explode in the microwave.

2) Microwave on HIGH for about 10 minutes, or until the potato is tender when you squeeze it.

3) Take out of the oven.

4) Microwave 1/2 cup of frozen broccoli (or other frozen vegetable) for about 2 minutes.

5) Split the potato, top with salt, pepper, the broccoli and some shredded cheddar cheese.

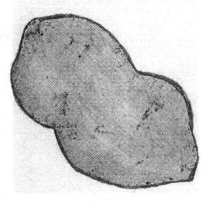

Main Dishes & Vegetables

Beyond Rice Cakes

Baked Sweet Potato

1 medium size sweet potato
Salt to taste
Margarine or butter, to taste
Brown sugar, to taste

1) Poke several holes in the potato.

2) Microwave for 8 to 10 minutes, or until it is tender when you squeeze it.

3) Season with salt, add some butter and enjoy.

4) If you are in the mood for something sweet, sprinkle brown sugar on top.

Main Dishes & Vegetables

Oven Roasted Potatoes

4 large brown potatoes
Vegetable oil
Onion powder
Garlic powder

1) Preheat oven on broil setting.

2) Slice potatoes into small round pieces.

3) Spread out on foil-lined baking tray.

4) Coat with thin layer of vegetable oil.

5) Sprinkle onion and garlic powder on top.

6) Bake until golden brown and crispy (about 15 minutes).

Main Dishes & Vegetables

Beyond Rice Cakes

Whipped Sweet Potato Bake

3 cans (15 oz) sweet potatoes, drained
1/4 cup (1/2 stick) butter or margarine, melted
1 teaspoon cinnamon
1/2 teaspoon salt
1/4 teaspoon ground nutmeg (optional)
3 cups miniature marshmallows

1) Place all ingredients except marshmallows in a medium bowl.

2) Beat with electric mixer on medium speed until well blended, or mash with a fork or potato masher.

3) Spoon into lightly greased microwavable 1-1/2 quart dish.

4) Microwave on HIGH for 8 to 10 minutes or until heated through, stirring after 5 minutes.

5) Top with marshmallows; let stand 2 to 3 minutes or until marshmallows begin to melt.

**OPTIONAL: place casserole under a hot broiler for one minute to brown the topping.

Main Dishes & Vegetables

Indian Corn Pudding

2 Tablespoon olive oil
1 medium red onion, chopped
1 red bell pepper, diced
1 1/2 cups fresh or frozen corn kernels (if using frozen, thaw before using)
3/4 cup grated cheddar cheese
1/2 cup low-fat milk
3 eggs, beaten
1/2 teaspoon dried basil or 1 Tablespoon chopped fresh basil
Salt and freshly-ground black pepper, to taste

1) Preheat oven to 350 degrees.

2) Grease a 1 1/2-quart shallow casserole dish or a 9-x 2-inch baking dish.

3) Heat the oil in a skillet and add the onions and red pepper.

4) Sauté for 5 minutes.

5) Remove from heat and place in a medium-sized bowl.

6) Add corn, cheddar cheese, milk, eggs, basil, and salt and pepper to taste.

7) Pour into the prepared casserole and bake for 30 minutes, or until a knife inserted in the center comes out clean.

Main Dishes & Vegetables

Beyond Rice Cakes

Baked Chicken Pasta Salad

1 (8 oz) pkg gluten-free penne pasta (rice pasta works best)
2-3 cups baked chicken (leftovers work great!!)
1 small zucchini chopped
1 bunch celery chopped
1 small red pepper chopped
3/4 cup gluten-free ranch salad dressing
1/4 cup freshly grated parmesan cheese, grated

1) Boil water in medium-sized sauce pan

2) Cook pasta.

3) Mix all ingredients together in large salad bowl.

4) Chill for about 20 minutes before serving.

5) This is great for bringing to a picnic!!

Main Dishes & Vegetables

Rice Pilaf

1 cup white rice
2 cups water
2 green onions, chopped
1 Tablespoon chopped parsley
2 grated carrots
1 teaspoon lemon juice
Dash of salt
Dash of pepper

1) Bring water to a boil on high heat.

2) Add the other ingredients.

3) Lower heat, simmer for 20 minutes, or until water is absorbed by the rice.

**OPTIONAL: You can also substitute grated zucchini and grated mushrooms if preferred.

Main Dishes & Vegetables

Beyond Rice Cakes

Tortilla Lasagna

1 (24 oz) can tomato sauce
1 cup onion chopped
1/4 teaspoon garlic powder
1 can refried beans
1 can black beans
1/2 teaspoon oregano
Cheddar cheese
Corn tortillas

1) Preheat oven to 375 degrees.
2) Spray 9 x 13-inch baking pan with non-stick spray.
3) Spread 1/4 cup of tomato sauce on bottom of pan.
4) In bowl combine remaining tomato sauce with onion, oregano and garlic powder.
5) Begin layering lasagna in the following order:

> Tortillas
> Beans
> Sauce
> Cheese
> Tortilla
> Beans
> Sauce
> Cheese

6) Cover and bake for 20 minutes.
7) Uncover and bake an additional 15 minutes.
8) Garnish with guacamole, sour cream and corn chips.

**OPTIONAL: can add layers of ground beef or turkey, as well as grilled vegetables for a more hearty lasagna

Main Dishes & Vegetables

Grandma's Noodle Kugel
In loving memory of Sarah Singer

1/2 stick butter or margarine

1/2 pound gluten-free twisty noodles

3 eggs

1 small carton cottage cheese

1/2 cup sour cream

2 teaspoon sugar

2 teaspoon cinnamon

1/3 cup raisins

3 cups milk

1) Preheat oven to 375 degrees.
2) Melt butter or margarine in baking pan.
3) Cook noodles. Drain.
4) Separate 3 eggs and beat yolks, reserving egg whites.
5) In a separate bowl, whip egg whites until stiff.
6) Combine noodles with egg whites, cottage cheese, sour cream, sugar, cinnamon and raisins in baking pan.
7) Stir in milk.
8) Fold in egg yolks.
9) Bake 60 minutes.

Main Dishes & Vegetables

Beyond Rice Cakes

Hush Puppies

2 cups cornmeal
1 teaspoon salt
2 teaspoon baking powder
1/2 cup grated onion
2/3 cup milk
1 egg
2 Tablespoon vegetable oil

1) Stir together cornmeal, salt, baking powder, onion, milk and egg.

2) Heat 2 Tablespoon vegetable oil or bacon grease in a frying pan on medium heat.

3) Dip large spoonfuls of cornmeal mixture into the oil and fry, turning with tongs, until outside is crispy.

Tips: Do not make dough balls too thick to ensure that they will cook evenly. Also, you might need to add more oil as you cook more dough balls.

Main Dishes & Vegetables

Swiss Vegetable Medley

1 bag each: frozen broccoli, carrots and cauliflower thawed and drained
1 can gluten-free cream of mushroom soup
1 cup shredded Swiss cheese
1/3 cup sour cream
1/4 teaspoon ground black pepper
1 jar (4 oz) chopped pimento, drained (optional)

1) Preheat oven to 350 degrees.

2) Combine vegetables, soup, 1/2 cup cheese, sour cream, pepper and pimento.

3) Pour into a 1-quart casserole.

4) Bake, covered with foil, for 30 minutes.

5) Top with remaining cheese.

6) Bake, uncovered, for 5 more minutes.

Main Dishes & Vegetables

Beyond Rice Cakes

Green Bean Casserole

2 (8 oz) cans green beans
1 can gluten-free cream of mushroom soup

1) Preheat oven to 400 degrees.

2) Combine green beans and soup in small casserole dish.

3) Bake for 25 minutes.

Main Dishes & Vegetables

Tomato & Rice Soup

1 can gluten-free tomato soup
1 cup medium grain white rice

1) Cook rice in rice cooker or on stove.

2) Stir soup and cooked rice together in saucepan.

3) Allow to simmer for about 5 minutes on medium heat.

4) Serve hot.

Main Dishes & Vegetables

Beyond Rice Cakes

Cheesy Cauliflower

1 head cauliflower
1 cup cheddar cheese

1) Chop cauliflower into bite-size pieces.

2) In microwavable dish sprinkle cheddar cheese over cauliflower.

3) Microwave on HIGH for 4 to 5 minutes.

4) Serve hot.

Main Dishes & Vegetables

Crustless Broccoli & Ham Quiche

3 large eggs
1 cup broccoli florets
1 cup ham, cubed
1 cup cream
1/2 cup Swiss cheese, shredded

1) Preheat oven to 375 degrees.

2) In small mixing bowl combine eggs and cream.

3) Slowly stir in all remaining ingredients.

4) Grease pie dish and pour mixture in.

5) Bake 25 minutes or until quiche is set.

Main Dishes & Vegetables

Beyond Rice Cakes

Chicken Parmesan

4 boneless, skinless chicken breasts
3 Tablespoon freshly grated Parmesan cheese
1 1/4 cup spaghetti sauce
1 cup mozzarella cheese, shredded
Parsley, chopped, to taste

1) Preheat oven to 350 degrees.

2) Place chicken in greased baking dish.

3) In small bowl combine Parmesan cheese and spaghetti sauce and gently stir together.

4) Cover with foil.

5) Bake 30 minutes.

6) Remove foil and top with cheese and parsley.

7) Bake an additional five minutes to melt cheese.

Main Dishes & Vegetables

Homemade Macaroni & Cheese

1 (6oz) pkg gluten-free elbow macaroni
1/2 cup milk
1 teaspoon salt
2 cups cheddar cheese, shredded
1 cup water

1) Cook elbow noodles in saucepan as directed on package.

2) Rinse noodles and place back in saucepan.

3) Add milk and 1/2 cup water.

4) Bring to a boil and cook until most liquid is absorbed.

5) Reduce heat and stir in cheddar cheese.

6) Preheat oven to BROIL setting.

7) Place in oven until top browns.

Main Dishes & Vegetables

Beyond Rice Cakes

Lemon Soaked Broccoli

1 pound fresh broccoli spears
2 Tablespoon butter or margarine
2 Tablespoon fresh lemon juice
1/3 cup water
Salt, to taste
Pepper, to taste

1) Wash broccoli and chop into bite-sized pieces.

2) Place broccoli in bottom of greased baking dish (Make sure dish is microwave safe).

3) Add 1/3 cup water to the bottom of pan.

4) Cover dish with paper towel and microwave for five minutes on high.

5) Drain excess water off of broccoli.

6) In separate small bowl, combine butter or margarine, lemon juice, salt and pepper.

7) Microwave until butter is melted.

8) Pour lemon/butter mixture on top of broccoli and serve hot.

Main Dishes & Vegetables

Sautéed Spinach

1 bag fresh spinach
4 Tablespoon olive oil
2 Tablespoon fresh lemon juice
2 teaspoon minced garlic

1) Wash spinach and pat dry.

2) In skillet, heat olive oil and brown garlic.

3) Add in spinach and sauté for about 5 to 7 minutes.

4) Add lemon juice and allow to simmer for 3 to 4 minutes.

Main Dishes & Vegetables

Beyond Rice Cakes

Lemony Endive Salad
* *Submitted by Christina Pirello*

3-4 Belgian endive, bottoms trimmed, leaves removed
1 red onion, very thin half moon slices
3 Tablespoon extra virgin olive oil
Sea salt, to taste
Black pepper, to taste
Fresh lemon juice, to taste
1 teaspoon honey
6-8 oil-cured black olives, pitted

1) Place endive leaves and onion in a mixing bowl.

2) Whisk together oil, a generous pinch of salt, black pepper, lemon juice and honey until mixture is smooth.

3) Pour over endive and toss to coat.

4) Arrange dressed endive mixture on a serving platter.

5) Top with olives.

6) Serve at room temperature or chilled.

Main Dishes & Vegetables

Desserts

Easy Peanut Butter Cookies*
Peanut Butter Chewies
Peanut Butter S'mores*
Special Cereal Bars
Lemon Drops
Golden Pineapple
Chocolate Pudding Cake
Lemon Pudding Cake
Flourless Chocolate Cake
Chocolate Clouds*
Butterscotch Blooms
Muddy Buddies*
Crispy Treats*
Lemon Squares
Ice Cream Delights*
Coconut Crispies
Coconut Brownies
Microwave-Safe Brownies*
Crispy Strawberry Crème Brulee*
Berry Whip*
Mocha Cheesecake Pudding
Peanut Butter Chocolate Bars
Chocolate Dipped Macaroons*

Spiced Ginger Cookies
Cheesecake Pudding*
Truffles*
Plum Apple Sauce
Tuxedo Strawberries
Rocky Road Candy
White Chocolate Delights
Almond Shortbread*
Fudge Brownies
Butterscotch Brownie Bars
Peppermint Patties*
Vanilla Sponge Cake
Snickerdoodles
Basic Chocolate Frosting
Buttercream Topping
Cream Cheese Glaze
Peach & Blueberry Sundae
Apple Blueberry Cobbler
Chocolate Covered Grapes
Sweetie Pies
Butterscotch Blondees
Fresh Berries in Champagne Sauce

*Denotes very easy to make

Beyond Rice Cakes

Easy Peanut Butter Cookies
Submitted by Erin Smith

1 cup peanut butter
1 cup sugar
1 egg

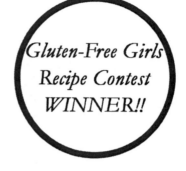

Gluten-Free Girls Recipe Contest WINNER!!

1) Preheat oven to 350 degrees.
2) Mix all ingredients together in medium sized mixing bowl.
3) Roll into 1-inch balls.
4) Place one inch apart on foil-lined cookie sheet.
5) Press with thumb or fork in crisscross pattern.
6) Bake 10 minutes.
7) Remove from oven and cool.

**OPTIONAL: Mix 3/4 cup of chocolate or butterscotch chips into the batter. Or, when cookies are almost baked, place a Hershey's kiss on each cookie. Put back in the oven, count to 10, and then take out and cool. Adding the chocolate is delicious!

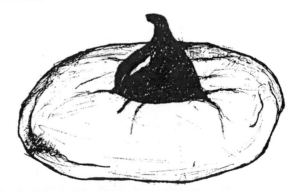

Desserts

Peanut Butter Chewies

1 cup peanut butter
1/2 cup brown sugar
2 Tablespoon honey
1/4 cup soy milk (can use whole milk)
5 teaspoon cornstarch

1)   Preheat oven to 325 degrees.

2)   Blend all ingredients together in medium-sized mixing bowl.

3)   Drop by teaspoonfuls onto ungreased baking sheet.

4)   Bake about 15 minutes.

5)   Take out of oven and put 3 to 4 chocolate chips into top of each cookie, slightly pressing in.

6)   Remove from pan and place on wire rack to cool.

Desserts

Beyond Rice Cakes

Peanut Butter S'mores

2 plain gluten-free frozen waffles
2 large marshmallows
4 squares of a chocolate bar
1 Tablespoon peanut butter

1) Toast gluten-free waffles to defrost.

2) Spread peanut butter over both waffles.

3) Place marshmallows and chocolate between two waffles and close like a sandwich.

4) Microwave on a plate for 30 seconds or until marshmallows and chocolate are melted.

5) Cut in half.

6) Serve with milk.

Desserts

Special Cereal Bars

6 cups gluten-free Chex type cereal (Health Valley Corn Crunch-Ems work well)
1 cup corn syrup
1 cup sugar
1 cup peanut butter

1) In medium-sized sauce pan, mix corn syrup, sugar and peanut butter together over medium heat.

2) Place 6 cups gluten-free cereal in large mixing bowl.

3) When syrup mixture begins boiling pour over top of cereal and mix until all cereal is coated.

4) Form into 3-inch balls and allow to harden on wax paper.

5) Serve with milk.

Desserts

Beyond Rice Cakes

Lemon Drops
*Submitted by Laura Moore

1 cup sugar
1/2 cup butter, softened
1/4 cup half & half
2 eggs
2 teaspoon grated lemon peel
1/2 teaspoon lemon extract
2 1/2 cups general purpose gluten-free flour
1 teaspoon baking powder
1/2 teaspoon salt

Glaze
1 cup powdered sugar
1-2 Tablespoon lemon juice

1) Heat oven to 350 degrees.
2) Combine sugar and butter in large bowl.
3) Beat at medium speed, scraping bowl often, until creamy.
4) Add half & half, eggs, lemon peel and lemon extract; continue beating until well mixed.
5) Reduce speed to low, add flour, baking powder and salt. Beat until well mixed.
6) Drop dough by rounded teaspoonfuls 2 inches apart onto parchment paper-lined cookie sheets.
7) Dip your finger into bowl of water and tap top of cookie to flatten slightly.
8) Bake for 10 to 12 minutes or until lightly browned. Cool completely.
9) Combine powdered sugar and enough lemon juice for desired glazing consistency in small bowl. Brush glaze onto cooled cookies with a pastry brush.

Desserts

Beyond Rice Cakes

Golden Pineapple

1 Pineapple
1/2 cup brown sugar
1 carton ice cream (vanilla ice cream or mango and coconut sorbet work best).

1) Preheat oven on BROIL setting.

2) With sharp kitchen knife cut skin off of pineapple.

3) Slice pineapple into 1-inch thick slices.

4) Arrange pineapple in small, individual-sized oven-safe baking dishes.

5) Sprinkle brown sugar on top.

6) Warm in oven until sugar melts and small bubbles form on top.

7) Top with scoop of favorite ice cream or sorbet.

Desserts

Beyond Rice Cakes

Chocolate Pudding Cake

1 1/4 cups sugar

1/2 cup white rice flour

1/2 cup soy flour

7 Tablespoon cocoa powder

2 teaspoon baking powder

1/4 teaspoon salt

1/2 cup milk

1/3 cup butter or margarine melted

1 1/2 teaspoon vanilla

1/2 cup light brown sugar packed

1 1/3 cup hot water

1) Preheat oven to 350 degrees.
2) In medium mixing bowl, combine sugar, flour, 3 Tablespoon cocoa, baking powder and salt.
3) Blend in milk, melted butter and vanilla. Beat until smooth.
4) Pour batter into square baking pan 8 x 8 x 2 inches.
5) In smaller bowl, combine remaining 1/2-cup sugar, brown sugar and remaining 4 Tablespoon cocoa.
6) Sprinkle mixture evenly over batter. Pour hot water over top. DO NOT STIR.
7) Bake 40 minutes. Let stand 15 minutes before serving.
8) Spoon into dessert dishes. Garnish with vanilla ice cream.

Desserts

Lemon Pudding Cake

3/4 cup sugar
1/2 cup white rice flour
1/2 cup soy flour
3 Tablespoon melted butter or margarine
1 teaspoon grated lemon peel
1/3 cup lemon juice
1 1/2 cups milk
3 eggs

1) Preheat oven to 350 degrees.

2) Combine sugar, flour and salt; stir in melted butter, lemon peel and lemon juice.

3) In separate bowl combine milk and well-beaten egg yolks.

4) Add to lemon mixture.

5) Fold 3 stiffly beaten egg whites into lemon mixture.

6) Pour into 8 x 8 x 2 inch baking pan.

7) Place pan in a larger 13 x 8-inch pan on oven rack.

8) Pour hot water into larger pan until 1 inch deep.

9) Bake for 40 minutes.

10) Serve warm or chilled.

Desserts

Beyond Rice Cakes

Stephanie's Flourless Chocolate Cake
Submitted by Stephanie Comeau

8 large eggs, cold
1 pound bittersweet chocolate or semisweet chocolate, coarsely chopped
1/2 pound unsalted butter (2 sticks), cut into 1/2-inch chunks
1/4 cup strong coffee or coffee-flavored liqueur (optional)
Confectioners' sugar or cocoa powder for decoration

1) Preheat oven to 325 degrees. Line bottom of 9-inch round pan with parchment paper and grease pan sides.

2) Cover pan underneath and along sides with sheet of heavy-duty foil and set in large roasting pan. Bring kettle of water to boil.

3) Beat eggs with hand-held mixer at high speed until volume doubles to approximately 1 quart, about 5 minutes.

4) Meanwhile, melt chocolate and butter (adding coffee or liqueur, if using) in large heat-proof bowl set over pan of almost simmering water, until smooth and very warm (about 115 degrees on an instant-read thermometer), stirring once or twice. (For the microwave, melt chocolate and butter together at 50 percent power until smooth and warm, 4 to 6 minutes, stirring once or twice.)

Continued…

Desserts

5) Fold 1/3 of egg foam into chocolate mixture using large rubber spatula until only a few streaks of egg are visible; fold in half of remaining foam, then last of remaining foam, until mixture is totally homogenous.

6) Scrape batter into prepared pan and smooth surface with rubber spatula. Set roasting pan on oven rack and pour enough boiling water to come about halfway up side of pan.

7) Bake until cake has risen slightly, edges are just beginning to set, a thin glazed crust (like a brownie) has formed on surface, and an instant read thermometer inserted halfway through center of cake registers 140 degrees, 22 to 25 minutes.

8) Remove cake pan from water bath and set on wire rack; cool to room temperature.

9) Cover and refrigerate overnight to mellow (can be covered and refrigerated for up to 4 days).

10) About 30 minutes before serving, invert cake on sheet of waxed paper, peel off parchment pan liner, and turn cake right side up on serving platter.

11) Sprinkle confectioners' sugar or unsweetened cocoa powder over cake to decorate, if desired.

12) Top with fresh or sugared fruit if desired.

Desserts

Beyond Rice Cakes

Chocolate Clouds

1 pkg instant chocolate pudding mix
2 cups milk
1 cup + 1 Tablespoon Cool Whip
1/8 cup fresh or frozen strawberries, raspberries or blueberries for garnish

1) In medium size mixing bowl, prepare pudding mix as directed on package with milk.

2) Once pudding has thickened, mix in one cup Cool Whip.

3) Spoon into serving dishes. For best results, freeze for 30 minutes before serving.

4) Top with small spoonful of Cool Whip and berries.

Desserts

Butterscotch Blooms

1 cup (2 sticks) butter or margarine
1 cup brown sugar
2 eggs
1 teaspoon vanilla
2 cups soy flour
1/4 cup rice flour
1 teaspoon baking soda
1/2 teaspoon salt
1 (12 oz) pkg butterscotch chips

**OPTIONAL: Add 1 heaping Tablespoon peanut butter (for extra moisture).

1) Preheat oven to 350 degrees.

2) In a large bowl, beat the butter, brown sugar, eggs and vanilla with an electric mixer.

3) Combine the flours, baking soda and salt, and gradually stir into the creamed mixture.

4) Mix in the butterscotch chips.

5) Drop by teaspoonfuls onto ungreased cookie sheets.

6) Bake for approximately 10 minutes.

Desserts

Beyond Rice Cakes

Muddy Buddies

9 cups gluten-free Chex type cereal (Health Valley Corn Crunch-Ems work well)
1 cup creamy peanut butter
1 cup chocolate chips
1 Tablespoon butter
1 teaspoon vanilla
1 box confectioners powdered sugar

1) Put the 9 cups of cereal in an extra-large bowl.

2) Combine the peanut butter, butter and chocolate chips in a microwavable bowl.

3) Heat in microwave on high for 1 minute, remove and stir. If not totally melted, heat for an additional 20 to 30 seconds more, but be careful not to burn the chocolate.

4) When totally melted, add vanilla and stir well.

5) Pour the chocolate over the cereal.

6) Stir with a rubber spatula until all the pieces are coated.

7) Pour the powdered sugar over the cereal.

8) With the spatula, stir the mixture until all the pieces are covered evenly with the sugar and not sticking together.

Desserts

Crispy Treats

6 cups Envirokids Koala Crisp cereal
1 pkg (10.5 oz) miniature marshmallows
4 Tablespoon butter or margarine
M & M's (16 oz pkg)

1) Microwave butter in a large microwavable bowl for 30 seconds, or until melted.

2) Add marshmallows and toss to coat.

3) Microwave on high for 1 minute and 20 seconds, or until marshmallows are completely melted and mixture is well blended, stirring after 45 seconds.

4) Add cereal IMMEDIATELY.

5) Toss in M&M's.

6) Mix lightly until well coated with the marshmallow mixture.

7) Press into greased 13-x 9-inch pan.

8) Cool completely. Cut into squares.

9) Wrap tightly in foil to keep fresh.

Desserts

Beyond Rice Cakes

Lemon Squares

3/4 stick butter
1 cup + 2 Tablespoon modified tapioca starch
1 cup granulated sugar
1/4 cup confectioner's sugar
2 eggs
2 Tablespoon lemon juice

1) Preheat oven to 350 degrees.

2) Mix butter, confectioner's sugar and 1 cup flour.

3) Press into pan and bake for 15 minutes.

4) Beat eggs, granulated sugar, 2 Tablespoon flour and lemon juice.

5) Pour over hot crust.

6) Bake 15 minutes.

7) Cut into squares when cooled.

8) Sprinkle with confectioner's sugar.

Desserts

Beyond Rice Cakes

Ice Cream Delights

Frozen Peanut Butter Cups
2 easy peanut butter cookies
1 scoop chocolate ice cream

Scoop ice cream onto flat side of one cookie. Place other cookie flat side down on top of ice cream. Squish down to make a sandwich.

Mint Chocolate Gummy Dream
2 scoops mint chocolate chip ice cream
1/2 cup gummy bears
1/2 cup hot fudge

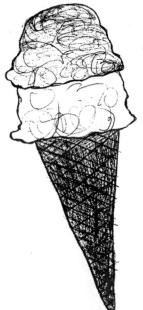

Mix gummy bears into ice cream until evenly distributed. Drizzle warm hot fudge and top with whipped cream and a cherry if desired.

Frozen Mocha Caramel Latte
2 scoops coffee ice cream
1/4 cup walnuts
1/4 cup chocolate chips
1/4 cup caramel sauce
1/4 cup hot fudge

Mix walnuts and chocolate chips into ice cream. Top with caramel sauce and whipped cream.

Desserts

Beyond Rice Cakes

Raspberry Rocky Road
2 scoops chocolate ice cream
1/4 cup miniature marshmallows
1/4 cup pecans
1/4 cup fresh raspberries
1/4 cup raspberry preserves

Mix all together and top with whipped cream.

Banana Blizzard
2 scoops vanilla ice cream
1 banana, sliced in thin slices
1/4 cup white chocolate chips
1/4 cup cool whip

Mix all together and eat immediately. To add color to this wintry mix, top with a cherry.

Classic Banana Split
1 banana
1 scoop each: chocolate, vanilla and strawberry ice cream
1/4 cup wet nuts
1/4 cup marshmallow sauce
1/4 cup hot fudge
1/4 cup frozen strawberry topping

Top sliced banana with all ingredients. Garnish with whipped cream and cherries.

Desserts

Coconut Crispies

1/3 cup powdered sugar
4 cups shredded coconut
6 egg whites
1 Tablespoon lemon juice
1 teaspoon vanilla flavoring
1/2 teaspoon almond flavoring
1/3 cup granulated sugar

1) Preheat oven to 300 degrees.

2) Mix all ingredients together in large mixing bowl.

3) Spoon tablespoon-sized balls onto greased baking pan.

4) Bake for about 45 minutes or until cookies are golden brown.

5) Cool before serving.

Beyond Rice Cakes

Coconut Brownies

1 cup almonds
1/2 cup sugar
6 Tablespoon cocoa powder
1/2 cup vegetable oil or margarine
2 eggs
1 cup coconut flakes

1) Preheat oven to 350 degrees.

2) Combine sugar, cocoa powder and oil in mixing bowl and set aside.

3) Beat eggs in separate bowl.

4) Stir sugar, cocoa powder and oil mixture into eggs.

5) Add almonds and coconut flakes.

6) Pour into greased pan.

7) Bake for about 10 minutes.

8) Cool before serving.

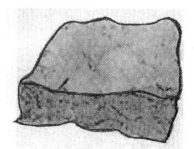

Desserts

Microwave-Safe Brownies

2 eggs
1cup sugar
1/2 teaspoon salt
1 teaspoon vanilla extract
1/2 cup melted butter (you may use cooking oil such as canola)
3/4 cup rice flour
1/2 cup cocoa powder
1/2 cup chopped walnuts
1/8 teaspoon peppermint extract

**Optional Peppermint Icing
2 Tablespoon butter
1 cup powdered sugar
1Tablespoon cream or milk
1/8 teaspoon peppermint extract

1) Beat together eggs, sugar, vanilla and salt.
2) Stir in rice flour, cocoa powder and nuts.
3) Spread batter in greased 10" glass baking pan.
4) For 700 watt microwave—bake on high for 5-6 minutes. For 1000 watt microwave bake for 6 minutes at 90% power.
5) Test with toothpick—the toothpick should come out of the brownies clean.
6) For icing, mix all ingredients together in mixing bowl and chill.
7) Drizzle icing over brownies before serving.

Desserts

Beyond Rice Cakes

Crispy Strawberry Crème Brulee

1 pkg fresh strawberries
1 cup vanilla yogurt
1/3 cup brown sugar

1) Preheat oven on BROIL setting.

2) Wash strawberries thoroughly and pat dry.

3) Slice strawberries lengthwise and arrange in small oven-safe dishes. (1 pkg of strawberries usually fits nicely into four small dishes).

4) Spoon about 1 Tablespoon of yogurt on top of each dish of straw-berries.

5) Top all dishes with brown sugar.

6) Place in oven until sugar melts.

7) Serve immediately.

Desserts

Berry Whip

1 pkg fresh or frozen blueberries
1 pkg fresh or frozen strawberries
1 pkg fresh or frozen raspberries
1 Tablespoon Cool Whip per serving prepared

1)   In medium bowl, gently stir together berries.

2)   Spoon into four small bowls.

3)   Top each with 1 Tablespoon of Cool Whip.

Desserts

Beyond Rice Cakes

Mocha Cheesecake Pudding

2 squares semi-sweet baking chocolate
1 Tablespoon butter or margarine
1 (8 oz) pkg softened cream cheese
1/3 cup sugar
1/3 cup instant mocha-flavored coffee
2 cups Cool Whip softened

1) In a small microwaveable-safe bowl, heat chocolate and butter on high for one minute.

2) Stir mixture until completely blended together.

3) In a separate bowl, beat sugar and cream cheese.

4) Gradually add-in flavored instant coffee to cream cheese blend.

5) Gently fold in Cool Whip.

6) Spoon pudding mixture into small serving bowls.

7) Drizzle chocolate mixture on top.

8) Top with small spoonful of Cool Whip.

Desserts

Peanut Butter Chocolate Bars

1/2 stick butter, softened
1 cup sugar
1/3 cup firmly packed brown sugar
1/2 cup milk
1/2 cup creamy peanut butter
1 egg
1 teaspoon vanilla
1 cup modified tapioca starch
1/2 teaspoon baking soda
1/4 teaspoon salt
3/4 cup mini semi-sweet chocolate chips

1) Preheat oven to 350 degrees.
2) Beat butter, sugar and brown sugar until well combined. Stir in milk, peanut butter, egg and vanilla until blended.
3) Gradually mix in gluten-free flour, baking soda and salt until blended.
4) Stir in chocolate chips.
5) Spread mixture evenly in well-greased 13 x 9-inch baking pan.
6) Bake for 25 minutes.
7) Cool completely in pan on wire rack.
8) Cut into squares.

Desserts

Beyond Rice Cakes

Chocolate Dipped Macaroons

1 (14 oz) pkg shredded coconut
2/3 cup sugar
6 Tablespoon all purpose gluten-free flour
4 egg whites
1 teaspoon almond extract
1 pkg semi-sweet chocolate chips

1) Preheat oven to 325 degrees.

2) Mix coconut, sugar, and flour in a bowl.

3) Blend in almond extract and egg whites.

4) Drop by spoonfuls onto greased and floured cookie sheets.

5) Bake for 20 minutes.

6) In separate bowl melt chocolate chips.

7) Partially dip macaroons in melted chocolate.

8) Refrigerate until chocolate solidifies.

Desserts

Spiced Ginger Cookies
Submitted by Sandy Chernow

3/4 cup butter
1 and 1/2 cups granulated sugar
1 beaten egg
1 teaspoon ginger
1 teaspoon cinnamon
1 small teaspoon cloves
1 teaspoon salt
2 teaspoon baking soda
4 Tablespoon dark molasses
1 cup rice flour
1 cup soy flour

1) Preheat oven to 375 degrees.

2) Cream butter and 1 cup of sugar.

3) Mix in other ingredients in given order.

4) Roll into small balls.

5) Roll the balls in the other ½ cup sugar.

6) Place 2 inches apart on cookie sheet.

7) Bake for 8 to 9 minutes or until light brown.

Desserts

Beyond Rice Cakes

Cheesecake Pudding

8 oz soft cream cheese
2 eggs
1/2 cup brown sugar
1 teaspoon almond flavoring
1/4 cup buttermilk

1) Preheat oven to 350 degrees.

2) Blend all ingredients together until creamy.

3) Spoon pudding into small baking dishes and bake for 20 minutes.

4) Refrigerate for about 1 hour before serving.

5) Garnish with fresh fruit.

Desserts

Truffles

4 oz soft cream cheese (plain or flavored)
6 Tablespoon cocoa powder
2 Tablespoon vegetable oil or margarine
1 teaspoon vanilla flavoring
2 cups powdered sugar

**OPTIONAL: 1 cup nuts or dried fruits if desired

1) Blend all ingredients together.

2) Add nuts or dried fruit last.

3) Roll into balls and chill in refrigerator for one hour before serving.

Desserts

Beyond Rice Cakes

Plum Apple Sauce
Submitted by Sylvia Chernow

1 lb small Italian plums
3/4 to 1 cup sugar, to taste
1/4 cup water
1 jar unsweetened apple sauce

1) Cut plums in half and remove seeds.

2) Combine halved plums, water and sugar in saucepan on medium heat until the plums are mushy and purple in color.

3) Stir plums into applesauce.

Desserts

Tuxedo Strawberries

1 cup white chocolate chips
1/2 cup semi-sweet or milk chocolate chips
2 cups strawberries

1) Line baking sheet with wax paper.

2) Melt white chocolate chips in dou-
    ble broiler or microwave. If using
    microwave, heat for 20-second
    increments and stir between heat-
    ing sessions until melted.

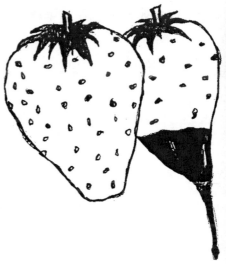

3) Be careful not to burn chocolate.

4) Dip strawberries in melted white
    chocolate, covering them almost
    up to the stem. Place in freezer or
    refrigerator until chocolate solidifies.

5) Melt semi-sweet or milk chocolate chips.

6) Dip tips of white-chocolate strawberries in semi-sweet or milk
    chocolate.

7) Place on baking sheet and put in freezer or refrigerator until
    chocolate tips solidify.

Desserts

Beyond Rice Cakes

Rocky Road Candy

1 cup semi-sweet chocolate chips
1/4 cup miniature marshmallows
1/4 cup chopped pecans or walnuts
1/4 cup maraschino cherries

1) Line baking sheet with wax paper.

2) Melt chocolate chips in double broiler or microwave. If using microwave, heat for 20-second increments and stir between heating sessions until melted.

3) Be careful not to burn chocolate.

4) Add marshmallows, nuts, and cherries into melted chocolate.

5) Using tablespoon, spoon globs of mixture onto baking sheet.

6) Place baking sheet in freezer until candy solidifies.

Desserts

White Chocolate Delights

1 cup white chocolate chips
1/4 cup miniature marshmallows
1/4 cup chopped pecans or walnuts
1/4 cup maraschino cherries

1) Line baking sheet with wax paper.

2) Melt chocolate chips in double broiler or microwave. If using microwave, heat for 20-second increments and stir between heating until melted.

3) Be careful not to burn chocolate.

4) Add marshmallows, nuts, and cherries into melted chocolate.

5) Using tablespoon, spoon globs of mixture onto baking sheet.

6) Place baking sheet in freezer until candy solidifies.

Desserts

Beyond Rice Cakes

Almond Shortbread

1/2 cup cornstarch
1/2 cup confectioner's sugar
1 cup rice flour
3/4 cup butter
2 Tablespoon almond extract

1) Preheat oven to 300 degrees.

2) Stir cornstarch, sugar and rice flour together.

3) Add in butter.

4) Mix dough with hands until soft mixture forms.

5) Shape into one-inch balls and place on greased cookie sheet.

6) Flatten with a fork.

7) Bake for 20-25 minutes.

Desserts

Fudge Brownies

1 cup water
1 teaspoon vanilla extract
1/2 cup margarine
1 cup sugar
1 egg
1/2 cup cooked cream of rice cereal
4 Tablespoon unsweetened cocoa
1 teaspoon baking powder

**OPTIONAL: add in nuts or coconut for added flavor

1) Preheat oven to 350 degrees.
2) In saucepan, heat water and margarine until the mixture comes to a boil.
3) Add rice cereal to boiling water and allow to simmer for one minute.
4) Remove pan from heat and cover for about five minutes.
5) Stir in egg and vanilla.
6) In separate bowl, combine sugar, cocoa and baking powder.
7) Slowly stir in cereal mixture.
8) Pour batter into greased 8 x 8 x 2 baking pan.
9) Bake for 40 minutes.

Desserts

Beyond Rice Cakes

Butterscotch Brownie Bars

3/4 cup butter
3/4 cup cocoa powder
2 1/2 cups sugar
4 eggs
1 cup rice flour
1/2 cup soy flour
1/2 teaspoon baking powder
1/4 teaspoon salt
1 cup butterscotch chips

1) Preheat oven to 325 degrees.

2) In saucepan, melt butter and stir in cocoa (can use a microwave to melt together if you don't have a stove).

3) Allow to cool, then stir in eggs and sugar.

4) Cream together and then add in all other ingredients.

5) Bake 20 minutes in 9-x 13-inch baking pan.

Desserts

Peppermint Patties

1/2 cup corn syrup
2 teaspoon peppermint extract
1/2 cup softened butter
6 cups confectioner's powdered sugar

**OPTIONAL: add two drops of food coloring

1) Combine corn syrup, butter and peppermint extract and add in sugar slowly.

2) Stir until smooth.

3) Shape mixture into one-inch balls and place on waxed paper.

4) Flatten each ball into a patty shape.

5) Let sit for about two hours before serving.

Desserts

Beyond Rice Cakes

Vanilla Sponge Cake

4 Tablespoon butter

3 eggs

1 cup rice flour

2 cups sugar

3 Tablespoon cornstarch

1 cup gluten-free vanilla-flavored soy milk

1 Tablespoon baking powder

1 Tablespoon vanilla extract

1) Preheat oven to 350 degrees.

2) Combine butter, eggs and sugar, and stir until creamy.

3) Add rice flour, cornstarch, vanilla extract and soy milk, and mix for about two minutes.

4) Add baking powder and stir until mixture is foamy.

5) Bake for about 40 minutes in greased pan.

Desserts

Snickerdoodles
In loving memory of Lela Mae Beach

1 cup margarine, softened

2 cups sugar

2 eggs

1/4 cup milk

1 teaspoon vanilla

2 cups rice flour

1 1/2 cups soy flour

1/2 teaspoon baking soda

1/2 teaspoon cream of tartar

1/2 teaspoon salt

Cinnamon-sugar, to taste

1) Preheat oven to 375 degrees.
2) In mixing bowl, cream margarine and sugar until light and fluffy.
3) Stir in eggs, one at a time, beating well after each.
4) Blend in milk and vanilla.
5) In separate bowl, thoroughly stir together gluten-free flour, baking soda, cream of tartar and salt.
6) Stir into creamed mixture.
7) Form dough into 1-inch balls.
8) Roll each ball in the cinnamon-sugar mixture.
9) Place balls 2 inches apart on greased cookie sheet.
10) Bake cookies about 10 to 12 minutes or until tan colored.

Desserts

Beyond Rice Cakes

Basic Chocolate Frosting

1/4 cup butter or margarine
1/4 cup milk
1 cup milk chocolate chips
1 teaspoon vanilla extract
2 3/4 cups powdered sugar

1) In a small saucepan, combine milk and butter.

2) Bring to a boil and then remove from heat.

3) Stir chocolate chips into milk and butter mixtures.

4) Slowly mix in vanilla extract and powdered sugar.

5) Mix until frosting is of a spreading consistency. You may need to add extra milk.

Desserts

Buttercream Topping

1/4 cup butter or margarine, softened
1 teaspoon vanilla extract
3 cups powdered sugar
4 Tablespoon milk

1) In small bowl cream butter until smooth and easily stirred.

2) Slowly add in vanilla, powdered sugar and milk.

3) Mix until mixture is creamy, adding milk by the teaspoon if necessary.

Desserts

Beyond Rice Cakes

Cream Cheese Glaze

1 (8oz) pkg cream cheese
1/2 cup butter or margarine, softened
1 teaspoon vanilla extract
1 (16 oz) box powdered sugar

1) Using a hand-held mixer, whip cream cheese until it reaches a smooth consistency.

2) Slowly add in butter and vanilla.

3) Last, slowly sift in powdered sugar and mix until smooth.

Desserts

Peach & Blueberry Sundae

2 cups fresh blueberries
4 peaches (white peaches work best)
1/8 cup sugar
1 pint vanilla ice cream

1) In medium size bowl sprinkle sugar on top of blueberries.

2) Allow blueberries to sweeten for about 30 minutes.

3) Place blueberry and sugar mixture in blender and mix until smooth.

4) Slice peaches and arrange in bottom of ice cream dish.

5) Place one scoop of vanilla ice cream on top of peaches.

6) Top ice cream with blueberry mixture.

Desserts

Beyond Rice Cakes

Apple Blueberry Cobbler

5 large apples, peeled and sliced
1 cup frozen blueberries
1 1/2 teaspoon cinnamon sugar
3/4 cup white rice flour
1 cup sugar
1/3 cup butter or margarine

1) Preheat oven to 350 degrees.

2) Line apples along the bottom of a greased baking dish.

3) Evenly distribute blueberries on top of apples.

4) Sprinkle 1/2 teaspoon cinnamon sugar on top of fruit.

5) In a separate mixing bowl combine remaining cinnamon sugar, rice flour, and sugar.

6) Using two knifes, cut butter or margarine into mixture.

7) Sprinkle mixture on top of fruit.

8) Bake 50 minutes.

Desserts

Chocolate Covered Grapes

4 bars white or milk chocolate
1 bunch of green grapes

1)   Separate grapes into small clusters.

2)   In small saucepan melt chocolate.

3)   Dip grape clusters into chocolate mixture.

4)   Allow to dry on wax paper.

5)   Place in refrigerator for about one hour before serving.

Desserts

Beyond Rice Cakes

Sweetie Pies

1 bag large marshmallows
1/2 cup butter or margarine
1 teaspoon vanilla extract
1 1/2 teaspoon pink food coloring
4 cups Health Valley Corn Crunch-Ems
1 cup M&M's

1) In a medium-sized saucepan melt marshmallows and butter, stirring constantly.

2) Stir in vanilla extract and food coloring.

3) Remove from heat and stir in cereal and M&M's.

4) Form into palm-sized balls and allow to harden on wax paper.

Desserts

Butterscotch Blondees

2 teaspoon butter or margarine
3 cups butterscotch chips
1 cup peanut butter
3 cups Health Valley Corn Crunch-Ems

1) In medium-sized saucepan, melt butter or margarine, butterscotch chips and peanut butter.

2) Remove from heat and stir in Corn Crunch-Ems.

3) Form into 2-inch balls and line on wax paper.

4) Chill before serving.

Desserts

Beyond Rice Cakes

Fresh Berries in Champagne Sauce
Submitted by Christina Pirello

10-12 fresh strawberries, rinsed well, stems removed, halved

Champagne Sauce:
1 cup champagne
1 pinch sea salt
2 Tablespoon honey
1 orange worth of zest
Handful of fresh mint sprigs

1) Arrange strawberry halves on a plate and chill separately.

2) While the berries chill begin making the sauce.

3) Combine champagne, salt, honey and orange zest in a small sauce pan and place over medium heat.

4) Cook, uncovered until the sauce reduces to a thick syrup.

5) Spoon sauce onto four individual serving plates.

6) Pile strawberries on top.

7) Serve garnished with mint sprigs.

Desserts

Gluten-Free Mixes

So you don't like to cook?? That's ok, not everyone loves to stand over a hot stove or wait for a luscious dessert to bake in the oven.

For those celiacs looking for pre-made gluten-free foods and mixes that are ready-to-eat or require very few ingredients, below is a list of some the tastiest options.

Gluten-Free Pantry

www.glutenfree.com

Favorite Sandwich Bread
Country French Bread—*great for pizza*
French Bread & Pizza Mix
Tom's Light Gluten-Free Bread Mix
Light Rye-Style Bread Mix
Dairy-Free Sandwich Bread Mix
Delicious Slicing Bread
Tapioca Bread Mix
Bagel Mix
Cranberry Orange Quick Bread and Muffin Mix
Orange Almond Biscotti
Buttermilk Brown Rice Pancake Mix
Muffin & Scone Mix

Quick Mix—*great for making crustless quiche and other quick dishes*

Beth's All-Purpose G-F Baking Flour

Blueberry Buckwheat Muffin & Pancake Mix

Harvest Pumpkin Quick Bread Mix

Apple Spice Quick Bread Mix

Bran Muffin Mix

Banana Quick Bread Mix—*makes banana bread or yummy banana pancakes—add choc chips, too*

Yankee Cornbread Mix—*add cheese, corn and salsa for a feast that everyone will love*

Old Fashioned Cake & Cookie Mix

Chocolate Truffle Brownie Mix—*it doesn't get easier or yummier than this*

Danielle's Chocolate Cake Mix

Coffee Cake Mix

Crisp & Crumble Mix

Chocolate Chip Cookie Mix

Spice Cake & Gingerbread Mix

Angel Food Cake Mix

Perfect Pie Crust Mix

Herb-Flavored Rice Crumb Coating

Pamela's Products

www.pamelasproducts.com

Butter Shortbread

Chunky Chocolate Chip Cookies

Chocolate Chip Walnut Cookies

Ginger Cookies

Lemon Shortbread

Peanut Butter Cookies

Pecan Shortbread

Shortbread Swirl
Ultimate Baking & Pancake Mix
Irresistible Chocolate Brownie Mix
Luscious Chocolate Cake Mix
Incredible Chocolate Chunk Cookies

Gluten-Free Cookie Jar

www.glutenfreecookiejar.com

Plain Bagels
Sesame Bagels
Poppy seed Bagels
Cinnamon Raisin Bagels
Pumpernickel Bagels
Pita Bread
Soft Pretzels
Brownies
Blueberry Scones
Chocolate Chip Cookies
Brown Sugar Wafers
Orange Chiffon Bundt Cake
Iced Chocolate Bundt Cake
White Bread Mix
Pita Bread Mix
Donut Mix
Cornbread Muffin Mix
Blueberry Muffin Mix
Banana Bread Mix
Pumpkin Bread Mix
Buttermilk Pancake Mix

Sun Flour Baking Company
www.sunflourbaking.com

Double Chocolate Cookies
California Bars
Cinnamon Twist Cookies
Chocolate Chip Cookies
Peanut Butter Cookies
Pumpkin Spice Cookies
Mint Chocolate Chip Cookies
German Chocolate Cookies

Whole Foods Market
www.wholefoods.com

Cinnamon Raisin Bread
Cornbread
Pizza Crust
Prairie Bread
Sandwich Bread
Sundried Tomato & Roasted Garlic Bread
Blueberry Muffins
Cherry Almond Streusel Muffins
Cream Biscuits
Almond Scones
Cranberry Orange Scones
Chocolate Chip Cookies
Molasses Ginger Cookies
Peanut Butter Cookies
Walnut Brownies

Banana Bread
Carrot Cake
Apple Pie
Cherry Pie
Pecan Pie

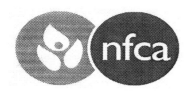

National Foundation for Celiac Awareness

The National Foundation for Celiac Awareness (NFCA), a nonprofit, was formed in 2003 by Alice Bast, a celiac sufferer who channeled her frustration and loss—including a full term stillbirth—into raising awareness and eventually funding research for a cure. Alice, along with many others, believe that the puzzle of autoimmunity can be solved by studying celiac disease, since it is the only autoimmune disease where the trigger—gluten—is known. Alice has assembled an influential Board of Directors and a renowned Medical Advisory Board who together will raise awareness and funds for research for this debilitating yet easily treatable disease.

Mission:

Our primary mission is to raise awareness of celiac disease among the public and the medical community. Our goal is simple: to gain a prompt and correct diagnosis for all Americans who have celiac disease. The Foundation's mission is to raise awareness and funding for celiac disease that will advance research, education and screening, and improve the quality of life of children and adults affected by this autoimmune disease through grant making and direct programming.

We envision a world in which:

- Celiac disease is widely recognized as one of the most common hereditary diseases.

- Better, more accurate and cost-effective screening methodologies available and in use.

- A pharmaceutical cure is in place to prevent the onset or mitigate the effects of this autoimmune disorder so that men and women suffering from celiac disease and dermatitis herpetiformis can lead a normal life.

NIH Consensus Development Conference on Celiac Disease:

The National Institutes of Health (NIH) has confirmed the beliefs of NFCA. Major developments came out of the NIH Celiac Disease Consensus Development Conference in June 2004. The following are some of the most dramatic:

1. Celiac disease has been reclassified. Once thought to be a rare childhood disease, it is now classified as a common disease that can affect people of all ages.

2. Celiac disease affects 1% of the population, about 3 million people in the United States.

NIH Recommendations:

1. Heightened awareness of celiac disease among general public.

2. Education of physicians, registered dieticians and other health care professionals to increase diagnosis.

3. Formation of a federation of celiac disease societies, celiac disease interest groups, individuals with celiac disease and their families, physicians, dieticians, and other health care providers.

4. Standardizations of serologic tests and pathologic criteria for the diagnosis of celiac disease.

5. Adoption of a standard definition of a gluten-free diet based on objective evidence.

6. Development of an adequate testing procedure for gluten in foods and definition in standards for gluten-free foods in the United States to lay the foundation for food labeling.

For more information:
www.celiaccentral.org

About the Author

Vanessa Maltin was born and raised in Hillsborough, Calif. She received a bachelor's degree in journalism from the George Washington University in May 2005 and is attending graduate school at Georgetown University. Currently, Vanessa is working with the National Foundation for Celiac Awareness to raise awareness about celiac disease and coordinate campaigns that seek to improve the lives of celiacs nationwide. Previously, she worked as a health care reporter for the Advisory Board Company's *Daily Briefing* and was a reporter for *Cox Newspapers* where she covered health care, politics, immigration and other breaking news for major daily newspapers including the *Palm Beach Post*, the *Atlanta Journal-Constitution*, the *Dayton Daily News* and the *Austin American Statesman*. She also served as the Washington, D.C. bureau chief and editor of *U-WIRE* and interned at CNN, the Campaign for Tobacco-Free Kids, CarryOn PR and for Rep. E. Clay Shaw Jr. from Florida. Her family now lives in Jupiter, Florida.

Thank You!!

Thank you to everyone who assisted me with this book. I could not have done it without you!!

Connie Maltin
Alan Maltin
Stacey Maltin

Julie Hyman and Amanda Mangalavite for their gorgeous artwork

The National Foundation for Celiac Awareness

Christina Perillo

Susan Schurr

Lee Tobin

Beth Hilson

Ann Whelan & *Gluten-Free Living*

Jesse B Rauch and the third grade class at Ruth K. Webb Elementary School

Diana Hocker, Elyse Eisenberg and the Advisory.com News staff at the Advisory Board Company for always volunteering to be fearless taste testers

Kate Ackerman, Lisa Blubaugh, Julie Hyman and Laura Kammerer for proof reading, editing and always being willing to offer advice on how to properly use commas

And everyone else who contributed to making this book a success!!